HEALING FROM TRAUMA

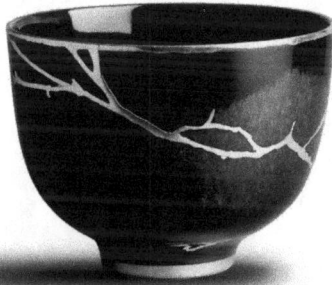

Reclaiming your Life

HEALING FROM TRAUMA

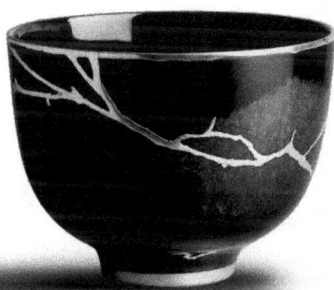

Reclaiming your Life

MAZDAK EBRAHIMI

Healing From Trauma: Reclaiming Your Life
1st Edition. 2024 v3.3

ASIN: B0DFLT4G2V (Amazon Kindle)
ISBN: 978-1-923223-11-0 (Amazon) PAPERBACK
ISBN: 978-1-923223-12-7 (Amazon) HARDCOVER
ISBN: 978-1-923223-13-4 (Ingram Spark) PAPERBACK
ISBN: 978-1-923223-14-1 (Ingram Spark) HARDCOVER
ISBN: 978-1-923223-15-8 (Smashwords)

CONTACT THE AUTHOR:
Author Website: www.mazdak.co

Table of Contents

❧

To my father and mother, whose boundless love and sacrifices have been the unwavering light guiding me through every step of my life. Thank you for giving me the strength to dream, the courage to pursue, and the heart to believe in myself. I owe everything to you.

To the steadfast soul who has accompanied me through every success and struggle, whose abiding presence has been my anchor in a shifting world. Patiently you provided avenues of reflection, inspiring strength and assurance when I needed them most.

With profound gratitude, I thank all my mentors and motivators whose influence has been the heartbeat of this book.

Your unwavering support has not only shaped this book but has forever touched my heart and soul in ways words can hardly express.

Unlock a deeper level of healing with our exclusive book bonuses!

As a valued reader of Healing From Trauma: Reclaiming Your Life, you're invited to access a set of transformative tools designed to support your journey.

These bonuses are crafted to help you actively engage with the techniques discussed in the book, making your healing process more interactive and personalised.

What You'll Get:

- **Guided Workbook/Journal**: Dive deeper into grounding techniques, breathing exercises, and processing trauma through narrative. This journal will guide you through reflective prompts and practical exercises, helping you apply what you've learned in the book to your own experiences.

- **Printable Mindfulness Exercises**: These easy-to-follow exercises are designed to keep you grounded and present. Perfect for daily practice, they'll help you maintain calm and focus in your everyday life.

- **Printable Affirmation Cards**: Reinforce positive thinking and self-compassion with these beautifully designed affirmation cards. Keep them handy for a daily boost of encouragement.

- **Downloadable Checklist for Finding Professional Help**: This comprehensive checklist guides you in choosing the right therapist or support professional, ensuring you find the help that best suits your needs.

These bonuses are available exclusively to our readers—don't miss out!

Visit *https://mazdak.co/page/resources*
to sign up and access your free bonuses today.

Introduction

Welcome to *Healing from Trauma: Reclaiming Your Life*, a book dedicated to providing support and guidance for individuals who have experienced trauma and are seeking to navigate the path toward healing and recovery. Trauma can have profound and lasting effects on our lives, impacting our mental, emotional and physical well-being. However, it is important to remember that healing is possible, and by understanding the nature of trauma and implementing effective coping strategies, you can regain control over your life.

Chapter 1 begins by establishing a foundation of knowledge regarding trauma. We will explore what trauma is and delve into different types of trauma, including acute, chronic and complex trauma. Understanding the various forms of trauma can help you identify and validate your own experiences and know you are not alone in your journey.

Chapter 2 focuses on recognising the signs and symptoms of trauma. Trauma can manifest in different ways, affecting our emotions, physical wellbeing and behaviours. By becoming familiar with the common symptoms associated with trauma, you can gain insight into your reactions and seek appropriate support.

In **Chapter 3**, we discuss coping strategies that can provide immediate relief in times of distress. These techniques – which include grounding exercises, deep breathing and progressive muscle relaxation – can help you manage overwhelming emotions and find a sense of calm amidst chaos. Additionally, we emphasise the importance of seeking support from your loved ones during challenging times.

Chapter 4 delves into the importance of seeking professional help when dealing with trauma. Therapists play a crucial role in guiding individuals through the healing process, and we explore different therapeutic approaches commonly used in trauma treatment, such as cognitive-behavioural therapy (CBT), eye movement desensitisation and reprocessing (EMDR), dialectical behaviour therapy (DBT), somatic experiencing (SE) and expressive therapies. This chapter also provides guidance on finding a qualified therapist to support your healing journey.

Chapter 5 introduces the concept of processing trauma through narrative. We explore the power of storytelling and the therapeutic benefits of journalling, writing your trauma narrative and embracing self-compassion and acceptance. Sharing your experiences and emotions in a safe and supportive environment can be a transformative step towards healing.

Chapter 6 focuses on building resilience and embracing post-traumatic growth. While trauma can be devastating, it is possible to develop resilience and find meaning and purpose in life again. We discuss the importance of self-care, nurturing healthy relationships and embracing personal growth and transformation.

In **Chapter 7**, we address trauma triggers and relapse prevention. Identifying triggers and developing strategies to manage them is crucial for maintaining stability and preventing setbacks during your healing journey. We also emphasise the significance of building a support network that understands and supports your ongoing recovery.

Chapter 8 concludes our ebook by emphasising the importance of moving forward and thriving after trauma. We discuss creating a new narrative and identity, setting realistic goals, and embracing self-compassion and forgiveness. Celebrating your progress and any small victories along the way is essential in fostering a positive outlook on your healing journey.

By exploring the chapters of this ebook, you will gain valuable insights and practical strategies, and you will receive the encouragement needed to navigate the complex path of healing from trauma. Remember, healing takes time, and every step forward is a step closer to reclaiming your life. Let's embark on this journey together, supporting one another as we find hope, resilience and a renewed sense of purpose.

About the Author

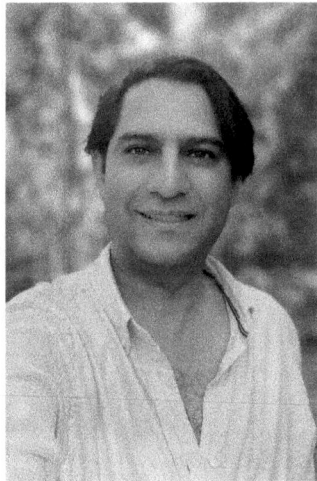

Mazdak Ebrahimi brings a unique perspective to the field of mental health and wellbeing, despite having no formal clinical credentials in psychology. Their insights are derived from personal experiences, providing a relatable narrative that will resonate deeply with readers navigating similar challenges.

Driven by a passion to offer hope, encouragement and guidance to those grappling with trauma and its aftermath, Ebrahimi embarked on this writing journey. Their narrative reflects resilience, courage and the transformative power of personal growth.

What distinguishes Ebrahimi is their willingness to confront trauma directly and explore the depths of their own psyche in search of healing and understanding. Through introspection, therapy and a commitment to self-discovery, they have emerged from the shadows of their past with newfound clarity and purpose.

Ebrahimi's narrative is refreshingly free from the jargon and technical language often found in academic literature, making *Healing From Trauma* accessible and relatable to a wide audience. Instead of relying on theoretical frameworks, they draw from their own experiences, offering practical insights and advice rooted in authenticity and empathy.

While this may be their first venture into mental health literature, Ebrahimi's voice is powerful and demands attention. Their willingness to share their insights with honesty and vulnerability is a testament to their courage and resilience.

Through their words, Ebrahimi offers solace, understanding and a guiding light for those embarking on their own journey of healing and self-discovery. As Ebrahimi's voice continues to evolve, they will undoubtedly become an even more potent force for change in the realm of mental health.

With each new chapter, they offer hope and inspiration to countless individuals struggling to find their way through the darkness. Their story is a reminder that no matter how daunting the journey may seem, there is always hope for healing and transformation.

Chapter One

Understanding Trauma

Trauma can have a profound impact on our lives, shaping our thoughts, emotions and behaviours. It disrupts our sense of safety and wellbeing, leaving lasting imprints on our minds and bodies.

Understanding trauma is a crucial first step towards healing and reclaiming our lives.

In this chapter we will explore the nature of trauma, its different types, and how it affects us on various levels.

1.1 What is Trauma?

Trauma is a complex and multifaceted experience that can impact an individual's life. It is important to understand what trauma is and how it differs from ordinary stress or adversity. In this section, we will explore the definition of trauma, its key features, and how it affects individuals on a psychological and physiological level.

Trauma can be defined as an event or series of events that overwhelm an individual's capacity to cope, causing a profound disruption in their sense of safety, control and wellbeing. It goes beyond the typical ups and downs of life, exceeding the individual's ability to adapt and process the associated emotions and sensations. While trauma is often linked to extreme events like natural disasters, accidents or violence, it can also result from ongoing situations, including abuse, neglect or prolonged exposure to stressful environments.

One key aspect of trauma is its subjective nature. What may be traumatic for one person may not be traumatic for another. Different individuals have unique backgrounds, vulnerabilities and resilience levels that influence how they perceive and respond to traumatic events. Trauma can be influenced by factors such as age, developmental stage, previous life experiences and available support systems.

Various criteria help distinguish trauma from everyday stress or adversity. Firstly, trauma tends to result from an unexpected or shocking event that disrupts an individual's sense of predictability and safety. Such events occur without warning, leaving the person feeling helpless and vulnerable. The intensity and severity of the event can significantly impact the degree of trauma experienced.

Secondly, trauma is characterised by the individual's subjective emotional response. It is not just the event itself that determines the level of trauma but also the emotional and psychological impact it has on the person. Common emotional responses to trauma include fear, helplessness, horror, guilt, shame and anger. These emotions may persist long after the traumatic event has ended and can influence the individual's thoughts, behaviours and overall wellbeing.

Another critical aspect of trauma is the disruption it causes to the individual's ability to function and engage in daily activities. Traumatic experiences can significantly impair cognitive functioning, memory, concentration and decision-making. Individuals may also experience difficulty regulating their emotions, which can lead to emotional dysregulation, mood swings and a sense of overwhelm.

It is important to note that trauma can have both immediate and long-term effects on an individual's wellbeing. Immediate reactions may include shock, denial, confusion or dissociation, while long-term effects can manifest as post-traumatic stress disorder (PTSD), depression, anxiety disorders, substance abuse and a range of physical health issues.

Trauma also affects individuals on a physiological level. When faced with a traumatic event, the body's stress response system, including the release of stress hormones like cortisol and adrenaline, becomes activated. This response is essential in preparing the individual to fight, flee or freeze in the face of danger. However, in the context of trauma, this response can become dysregulated, leading to long-term physiological imbalances. Chronic activation of the stress response system can result in sleep disturbances, compromised immune function, gastrointestinal issues and chronic pain.

In conclusion, trauma is a deeply distressing and overwhelming experience that disrupts an individual's sense of safety, control and wellbeing. It goes beyond ordinary stress or adversity, impacting individuals on psychological, emotional and physiological levels. Trauma is subjective, with different individuals responding to events in unique ways based on their backgrounds and vulnerabilities. By understanding the nature of trauma, we can begin to develop strategies and approaches that facilitate healing and support individuals to reclaim their lives.

1.2 Types of Trauma

Trauma manifests in many ways. This section will explore the differences between trauma types. their characteristics and the immediate effects along with the impacts it has psychologically and physically.

Acute Trauma

Acute trauma refers to a single traumatic event with a defined beginning and end. This type of trauma can occur unexpectedly, leaving a profound impact on an individual's life. Acute trauma can result from events such as natural disasters, car accidents, physical assault or witnessing violence.

In this section, we will explore the characteristics of acute trauma, its immediate effects and potential long-term consequences.

Characteristics of Acute Trauma

Often characterised by the suddenness and intensity of the event, acute trauma can happen in a matter of seconds or minutes, catching individuals off guard and disrupting their sense of safety. The traumatic event may involve a threat to one's life or physical integrity, or witnessing such threats happening to others. The intense emotions and sensations associated with acute trauma can be overwhelming, affecting the individual's ability to cope and process the experience effectively.

Immediate Effects of Acute Trauma

Immediately following an acute traumatic event, individuals may experience a range of reactions and responses. These can include shock, disbelief and emotional numbness. The body's fight-or-flight response may be activated, leading to increased heart rate, rapid breathing and heightened senses. Flashbacks, nightmares and intrusive thoughts about the traumatic event are also common. Individuals may exhibit signs of acute stress disorder (ASD), which shares similarities with post-traumatic stress disorder (PTSD) but occurs within the first month after the trauma.

Psychological Impact of Acute Trauma

The psychological impact of acute trauma can be significant and vary from person to person. Some individuals may develop symptoms of PTSD, which can include re-experiencing the traumatic event through flashbacks or nightmares, avoiding reminders of the trauma, experiencing negative thoughts and moods, and increased arousal or hypervigilance. Others may struggle with anxiety, depression, guilt, or even survivor's guilt where they question why they survived when others did not. These psychological effects can interfere with daily functioning, relationships and overall wellbeing.

Physical Impact of Acute Trauma

The body's response to trauma can manifest as physical symptoms, such as sleep disturbances, fatigue, headaches, muscle tension and gastrointestinal problems, all of which impact physical wellbeing. Some individuals may experience changes in appetite, weight or sexual function. In addition, the immune system can be compromised, making individuals more susceptible to illness and infections.

Long-term Consequences of Acute Trauma

While acute trauma is a single event, its effects can persist long after the event itself has ended. If not adequately addressed and treated, acute trauma can contribute to the development of chronic psychological conditions such as PTSD, anxiety disorders or depression. Individuals may experience difficulty trusting others, or may struggle with feeling vulnerable or unsafe. They may also develop maladaptive coping mechanisms, such as substance abuse, to manage their distress. It is crucial to seek support and appropriate treatment to minimise the long-term consequences of acute trauma.

Chronic Trauma

Chronic trauma is a form of trauma that involves exposure to traumatic events or stressful environments over an extended period. Unlike acute trauma, which is characterised by a single traumatic event, chronic trauma encompasses a sustained experience of trauma that can last for months, years or even a lifetime.

This section will delve into the nature of chronic trauma, its effects on individuals and strategies for coping and healing.

Understanding Chronic Trauma

Chronic trauma manifests in various forms and can stem from different sources. Common examples of chronic trauma include domestic violence, childhood abuse and neglect, and war and political conflict.

Domestic Violence

Living in a household where one experiences ongoing physical, emotional or sexual abuse can lead to chronic trauma. Repeated exposure to violence and fear can have severe consequences for an individual's wellbeing.

Domestic violence refers to the pattern of abusive behaviours that occur within a familial or intimate relationship, where one person seeks to exert power and control over another. Domestic violence is a deeply distressing and pervasive issue that affects individuals of all genders, ages, races and socioeconomic backgrounds, and may involve physical, emotional, psychological, sexual or financial abuse, or a combination of these.

Physical Abuse

Physical abuse is a form of domestic violence that involves the intentional use of force against a victim, resulting in physical harm or injury. It is a visible and tangible form of abuse, leaving physical marks and scars. Physical abuse can take various forms, ranging from mild to severe, and can include acts of hitting, punching, slapping, kicking, choking, burning, or using weapons. Physical abuse is often characterized by the abuser's desire to exert power and control over the victim. It is not limited to a specific gender, age, or cultural background and can occur in any intimate or familial relationship. The impact of physical abuse extends far beyond the immediate physical injuries, as it also leaves deep emotional and psychological scars.

The effects of physical abuse can include:

- *Physical Injuries*

Physical abuse often leads to a range of injuries, varying in severity. These injuries can include bruises, cuts, burns, broken bones, internal injuries and head trauma. The severity of the injuries depends on the force applied by the abuser and the areas of the body targeted. In some cases, physical abuse can result in long-term or permanent physical disabilities.

- *Emotional and Psychological Impact*

Physical abuse takes a significant toll on the victim's emotional and psychological wellbeing. Survivors may experience intense fear, anxiety and hypervigilance, where they are constantly anticipating and fearing the next violent episode. They may develop symptoms of PTSD, such as intrusive thoughts, nightmares and flashbacks related to the abusive incidents. The emotional impact of physical abuse often leads to low self-esteem, feelings of shame, guilt and self-blame.

- *Trauma and Mental Health Issues*

The trauma of physical abuse can contribute to the development of various mental health issues. Survivors may experience depression, anxiety disorders, substance abuse problems and suicidal thoughts. Long-term exposure to physical violence can create a sense of hopelessness, helplessness and a distorted view of self and the world around them.

- *Cycle of Violence*

Physical abuse is often part of a repetitive cycle of violence within an abusive relationship. The cycle typically includes a build-up of tension, followed by the occurrence of the abusive incident, and then a period of remorse or reconciliation. This cycle can create confusion. The abuser may express remorse, apologise or promise to change during the reconciliation phase, leading the victim to question their safety and the possibility of leaving the abusive relationship.

- *Impact on Children*

Children who witness physical abuse between their parents or caregivers experience profound emotional and psychological harm. They are at a higher risk of developing behavioural issues, experiencing difficulties at school and perpetuating the cycle of violence in their own relationships later in life. Witnessing physical abuse can leave long-lasting scars on a child's sense of security, trust and wellbeing.

There are ways to help individuals cope with physical abuse and heal:

- *Seek Support*

Reaching out for support from trusted individuals or organisations that specialise in domestic violence can be vital for survivors. Support groups, counselling services and helplines can provide emotional support, validation, information and resources to help navigate the healing process.

- *Trauma-Informed Therapy*

Engaging in trauma-informed therapy with a trained professional can assist survivors to process traumatic experiences, address emotional wounds and develop coping strategies. Therapeutic approaches, such as cognitive-behavioural therapy (CBT), dialectical behaviour therapy (DBT), or eye movement desensitisation and reprocessing (EMDR) can be effective in addressing the effects of physical abuse.

- *Self-Care and Self-Compassion*

Prioritising self-care activities that promote healing, self-nurturance and self-compassion is crucial. Engaging in mindfulness exercises, relaxation techniques, creative outlets and self-care rituals can help survivors reconnect with themselves and foster a sense of empowerment.

- *Building a Supportive Network*

Building a network of supportive and understanding individuals is essential for the healing journey. Surrounding oneself with trusted friends, family members, support groups or advocacy organisations can provide validation, understanding and assistance in rebuilding a sense of trust and security.

Remember, healing from physical abuse takes time and each survivor's journey is unique. It is important to seek professional help and support from those who specialise in domestic violence to ensure a comprehensive approach to healing and recovery.

Emotional and Verbal Abuse

Emotional and verbal abuse involves belittling, demeaning, insulting or constantly criticising the victim. The abuser may engage in gaslighting, manipulation and control tactics that erode the victim's self-esteem and sense of self-worth.

Emotional and verbal abuse are forms of chronic trauma that can have significant and long-lasting effects on an individual's mental and emotional wellbeing.

Let's explore these forms of abuse in more detail.

- *Emotional Abuse*

Emotional abuse involves a pattern of behaviours that are aimed at undermining an individual's self-worth, confidence and emotional stability. It often occurs in relationships where there is a power imbalance, such as intimate partnerships, parent-child relationships or even in professional settings. Some common examples of emotional abuse include:

- Humiliation and belittlement where the abuser may constantly criticise, mock or belittle the victim, undermining their self-esteem and self-worth. They may make derogatory comments, insulting their appearance, abilities or intelligence, and leaving the victim feeling small and inadequate.

- Gaslighting is a manipulative tactic used by abusers to make the victim doubt their reality and perception of events. They may distort or deny facts, manipulate the victim's memory or make them question their sanity or recall of events. This can leave the victim feeling confused, disoriented and unable to trust their own judgement.

- Isolation is a tactic emotional abusers often use to keep their victims away from friends, family and support systems. They may discourage or prevent the victim from engaging in activities or maintaining relationships outside of the abusive dynamic. This isolation can leave the victim feeling trapped, alone and reliant on the abuser for emotional support.

- Threats and intimidation are used by emotional abusers to control and manipulate their victims. They may threaten to physically harm themselves, the victim or loved ones, creating a constant atmosphere of fear and anxiety. This instills a sense of powerlessness and submission in the victim.

- *Verbal Abuse*

Verbal abuse involves the use of words, tone and language to demean, criticise and harm the victim. It can be overt or subtle, but its impact on the victim's emotional wellbeing is significant. There are several forms of verbal abuse.

- Insults and name-calling is the use of derogatory language to degrade and dehumanise the victim. Verbal abusers may attack the victim's character, intelligence, appearance or any other aspect they can exploit. This constant barrage of insults can erode the victim's self-esteem and sense of self-worth.

- Constant criticism is a relentless pattern of criticism, where the verbal abuser finds fault with everything the victim says or does. They may nitpick, berate or undermine the victim's abilities, decisions or achievements. Continuous criticism can leave the victim feeling inadequate, self-conscious and constantly on edge.

- Verbal threats are threats of violence, harm or abandonment that verbal abusers use to control and intimidate their victim. They instill fear and anxiety by making explicit threats to the victim's safety or wellbeing, or the safety of loved ones.

- Manipulative communication is the use of tactics that allow verbal abusers to control their victims. This may include using guilt, blame-shifting or twisting words to make the victim feel responsible for the abuser's actions or emotions. Abusers may also employ coercive language to force compliance or obedience.

The emotional and verbal abuse experienced in chronic trauma can have severe and long-lasting effects on individuals. Victims may develop symptoms of anxiety, depression, low self-esteem or self-doubt, and may struggle with trust and healthy relationships. It is crucial that survivors seek support and therapy, and that they develop strategies to heal from the effects of emotional and verbal abuse.

- *Psychological Abuse*

Psychological abuse targets the victim's mental and emotional wellbeing. It may involve threats, intimidation, isolation from family and friends, stalking or constant surveillance.

Psychological abuse is a form of chronic trauma that involves the use of words, actions or behaviours to manipulate, control and undermine an individual's sense of self-worth and wellbeing. It is often characterised by patterns of coercive control, humiliation, intimidation and emotional manipulation. Psychological abuse can occur in various settings, including personal relationships, workplaces and institutions. Understanding the impact and dynamics of psychological abuse is crucial for recognising and addressing this form of chronic trauma.

Psychological abuse can take many forms and its manifestations can vary widely. There are a number of patterns of psychological abuse.

- Verbal attacks involve the use of derogatory language, insults, name-calling or demeaning comments to belittle and degrade the individual. Verbal attacks can be explicit or subtle, and they are aimed at undermining the individual's self-esteem and creating a sense of powerlessness.

- Gaslighting is a manipulative tactic used to distort an individual's perception of reality and make them doubt their own experiences and sanity. It involves denying or minimising abusive behaviour, manipulating facts and making the victim question their memory, judgement and perception of events.

- Control and isolation are often used by psychological abusers to exert control over their victims and isolate them from friends, family and support networks. They may monitor their activities, control their finances, restrict their freedom and manipulate their social interactions to maintain power and dominance.

- Threats and intimidation are commonly used in psychological abuse. Threats, both explicit and implicit, are used to instill fear and maintain control. Threats may pertain to physical harm, harm to loved ones or consequences for non-compliance; in turn, these lead to the victim becoming intimidated.

- Emotional manipulation involves psychological abusers using tactics such as guilt-tripping, emotional blackmail, manipulation of affection or love and shifting blame to maintain power and control over their victims.

Psychological Impact of Psychological Abuse

Psychological abuse can have a profound and long-lasting impact on an individual's mental and emotional wellbeing. Let's look at come of the psychological consequences of psychological abuse.

- Low self-esteem and self-worth can be the result of constant criticism, humiliation and belittlement. Victims may internalise negative messages, develop a negative self-image, and struggle with feelings of shame, inadequacy and self-doubt.

- Anxiety and depression can be the result of the chronic stress and emotional turmoil caused by psychological abuse. Individuals may experience persistent feelings of fear, worry, sadness and hopelessness.

- Post-traumatic stress symptoms tend to be associated with PTSD. Flashbacks, intrusive thoughts, nightmares, hypervigilance and avoidance behaviours may occur as a result of the trauma endured.

- Self-blame and guilt are tactics often used by psychological abusers to manipulate victims into believing the abuse is their fault. This can further lead to a distorted sense of responsibility for the abusive behaviour, eroding self-esteem and any sense of agency they may have.

- Social and interpersonal challenges, including social withdrawal, difficulty trusting others and challenges in forming healthy relationships are often the consequence of the isolation and control exerted by psychological abusers. Individuals may struggle with boundaries, assertiveness and maintaining healthy connections with others.

Healing and Recovery

Healing from the psychological impact of abuse is a complex process that requires support, self-compassion and professional help. Strategies to support healing and recovery are important.

- Seeking professional support and working with a therapist or counsellor who specialises in trauma and abuse can provide essential guidance. Therapists can help individuals process their experiences, develop coping skills, rebuild self-esteem and address any mental health challenges.

- Establishing a safe environment and setting clear boundaries are essential when healing from psychological abuse. This may involve seeking legal protection, distancing oneself from the abuser and surrounding oneself with supportive and trusted individuals.

- Developing self-care practices that promote self-nurturance, relaxation and emotional wellbeing is vital. Activities may include journalling, meditation, engaging in hobbies, practising mindfulness and seeking out pleasurable experiences.

- Rebuilding self-esteem and self-identity are crucial to healing. This may involve challenging negative self-beliefs, practising self-compassion and engaging in activities that promote self-discovery and personal growth.

- Connecting with supportive networks and individuals who understand and validate one's experiences is essential. Support groups, therapy groups or online communities can provide a safe space for sharing, learning from others and fostering a sense of belonging.

To sum up, psychological abuse is a form of chronic trauma that can have significant and lasting effects on an individual's mental and emotional wellbeing. Recognising the patterns of psychological abuse and understanding its impact are essential in breaking free from the cycle of abuse and initiating the healing process. Seeking professional support, establishing safety and boundaries, practising self-care and connecting with supportive networks are vital steps towards recovery and reclaiming a sense of self-worth and agency.

Remember, healing is possible and you deserve a life free from abuse and filled with compassion and empowerment.

- *Sexual Abuse*

Sexual abuse within a domestic violence context includes non-consensual sexual acts, coerced sexual activities or any form of sexual degradation or humiliation.

Sexual abuse is a deeply traumatic experience that can have long-lasting effects on an individual's life. It involves any form of sexual activity or behaviour that is forced upon someone without their consent. When sexual abuse occurs repeatedly over a sustained period, it becomes a form of chronic trauma and can significantly impact a person's wellbeing.

Here, we will delve further into the effects of chronic sexual abuse and explore coping strategies for healing.

- *Effects of Chronic Sexual Abuse*

The effects of chronic sexual abuse can be profound and can manifest in various ways.

- The emotional and psychological impacts of chronic sexual abuse may include intense feelings of shame, guilt, fear and self-blame. Survivors may struggle with low self-esteem, self-destructive behaviours and a distorted sense of identity and sexuality. Additionally, they may develop symptoms of PTSD, anxiety disorders, depression and disassociation, and may have difficulty forming and maintaining healthy relationships.

- Trust and intimacy issues are common consequences of chronic sexual abuse. Survivors may struggle with establishing boundaries, expressing their needs and desires and distinguishing healthy, consensual relationships from abusive ones. Trusting oneself and others can be challenging and may require time, patience and therapeutic support.

- Body image and self-worth can be significantly impacted by chronic sexual abuse. Feelings of shame and self-blame can lead to a negative body image, and a sense of being damaged or unworthy. Healing from chronic sexual abuse often involves reclaiming ownership of one's body, rebuilding self-esteem and fostering self-acceptance.

- Sexual functioning and intimacy can be challenging for survivors of chronic sexual abuse. Challenges can range from difficulties with sexual desire, arousal or orgasm to experiencing pain or discomfort during sexual activity. Re-establishing a healthy and fulfilling sexual life often requires specialised therapeutic support to address these issues.

Coping and Healing Strategies

While healing from chronic sexual abuse can be a complex and individualised process, some strategies can provide support and aid in the journey to recovery.

- Seeking professional help and engaging in therapy with a trauma-informed therapist who specialises in treating survivors of sexual abuse is crucial. Therapists trained in trauma-focused approaches, such as CBT, DBT, or trauma-focused cognitive processing therapy (TF-CBT), can help survivors process their experiences, develop coping skills and work through the emotional and psychological impact of the abuse.

- Joining a support group and connecting with other survivors can offer validation, empathy and a sense of belonging. Sharing experiences, listening to the stories of others and receiving support from those who have walked a similar path can be immensely healing and empowering.

- Practising and prioritising self-care is crucial to aid healing from chronic sexual abuse. Activities such as journalling, meditation, creative expression, spending time in nature or engaging in hobbies and interests that bring joy and a sense of fulfillment can all help to promote self-nurturance, self-compassion and overall wellbeing.

- Establishing a safe environment and setting clear boundaries is essential for survivors of sexual abuse. This may involve implementing safety plans, developing assertiveness skills, learning to say no and surrounding oneself with trusted individuals who respect and support their boundaries.

- Exploring body-centreed therapies, such as somatic experiencing, can help survivors reconnect with their bodies, release stored trauma and regain a sense of safety and empowerment. These therapies focus on addressing the physical sensations and impacts of trauma, allowing survivors to heal on a holistic level.

- Engaging in self-exploration and educating oneself about sexual abuse, trauma and recovery can provide survivors with the knowledge and tools needed for their healing journey. Reading books, attending workshops or conferences and accessing online resources can empower survivors with information and help them make informed choices about their healing process.

Remember that healing from chronic sexual abuse takes time and patience. Each survivor's journey is unique and there is no one-size-fits-all approach. It is important to seek support, be gentle with oneself and surround oneself with caring individuals who can provide a safe and nurturing environment for healing. With the right support and resources, it is possible to reclaim a sense of control, rebuild trust and foster a fulfilling and empowered life beyond the impact of chronic sexual abuse.

- *Financial Abuse*

Financial abuse involves controlling the victim's finances and limiting their access to financial resources. The abuser may restrict the victim's access to money, withhold financial support or force them into economic dependence. Financial abuse is a form of chronic trauma that involves the control, manipulation or exploitation of an individual's financial resources by another person. It is often seen in the context of abusive relationships, where the abuser uses financial tactics to exert power and control over their victim.

Understanding Financial Abuse

Financial abuse can take various forms.

- Financial control occurs when the abuser restricts the victim's access to money, controls all financial decisions and withholds the funds necessary for basic needs. This may involve limiting access to bank accounts, denying access to income or forbidding the victim from working or pursuing education.

- Resource exploitation is when the abuser exploits the victim's financial resources for personal gain, often by coercing them into providing money or assets. This may include taking control of the victim's assets, coercing them to sign financial documents or stealing their money or property.

- Sabotaging employment or education undermines the victim's ability to gain financial independence. This may involve preventing the victim from attending work or school, damaging their professional reputation or interfering with their job search efforts.

- Accumulating debt in the victim's name, without their consent, can lead to financial burdens and damag to their credit rating. This can leave the victim responsible for repaying debts they did not incur, making it even more challenging for them to regain financial stability.

Effects of Financial Abuse

Financial abuse can have devastating consequences for victims.

- Financial dependence is fostered by the abuser when they control the victim's finances. This makes it difficult for the victim to leave the abusive relationship or assert their independence.

- Economic instability, where the victim may struggle to meet their basic needs, pay bills or maintain stable housing, is often the result of financial abuse. The lack of control over their financial resources can trap victims in a cycle of poverty and dependence.

- The emotional and psychological impact of constant manipulation and control exerted through financial abuse can be significant. Victims may experience feelings of distress, shame, guilt, powerlessness and low self-esteem. Financial stress can also lead to anxiety, depression and other mental health challenges.

- Barriers to leaving the abusive relationship are common and significant. The lack of financial resources, employment opportunities and access to credit can make it challenging to establish independence and escape the control of the abuser.

Coping and Healing Strategies:

Recovering from financial abuse requires a combination of practical and emotional strategies.

- Seeking financial support and resources is recommended. Reach out to organisations and resources that specialise in supporting individuals experiencing financial abuse. These organisations can assist with the creation of safety plans, accessing emergency funds and connecting with legal and financial professionals who can help navigate the complex financial aspects of abuse.

- Rebuilding financial independence by opening individual bank accounts, establishing credit in your name and developing a budget and savings plan is crucial. Individuals may consider seeking financial education or counselling to gain the knowledge and skills necessary for long-term financial stability.

- Emotional support and therapy is a key step. Engaging in therapy or support groups specifically tailored for survivors of financial abuse can provide validation, emotional support and guidance in healing from the trauma and rebuilding self-esteem and confidence.

- Self-care and self-empowerment activities can promote healing. This may involve engaging in activities that boost self-esteem, setting boundaries, practising self-compassion and cultivating a support network of trusted friends and family members.

Financial abuse is a form of chronic trauma that can have long-lasting effects on an individual's financial wellbeing and overall quality of life. Recognising the signs of financial abuse, understanding its impact and seeking support are crucial steps towards healing and regaining financial independence. Remember that you are not alone, and there are resources available to help you break free from the cycle of financial abuse and rebuild a life of security and empowerment.

Dynamics of Domestic Violence

Domestic violence is characterised by a cycle of abuse that often includes three phases: tension-building, acute abuse and honeymoon.

During the tension-building phase, tension and conflict escalate within the relationship. The victim may feel they are walking on eggshells as they fear that any action could trigger an outburst from the abuser.

The acute abuse phase is where the actual acts of abuse occur. The abuser may engage in physical, emotional or sexual violence, exerting power and control over the victim.

After the abusive episode, the honeymoon phase follows. During this phase, the abuser may display remorse by apologising or exhibiting behaviours aimed at reconciliation. This phase often involves promises to change, expressions of love and temporary periods of calm.

Impact of Domestic Violence

The effects of domestic violence on survivors can be severe and long-lasting. They may experience a wide range of physical, emotional and psychological consequences.

Physical injuries are common among victims of domestic violence, and may include bruises, fractures, internal injuries and chronic pain. These injuries may require medical attention and can have long-term health implications.

Emotional trauma is a significant consequence of domestic violence. Survivors often experience anxiety, depression, fear, PTSD and suicidal thoughts. The constant stress and fear created by the abusive environment can take a toll on mental wellbeing.

Survivors may develop low self-esteem and feelings of shame, guilt and self-blame. The abuser's manipulative tactics often lead victims to believe that the abuse is their fault or that they deserve it.

Isolation from family and friends is another consequence of domestic violence. Abusers employ tactics to control and isolate their victims, cutting off their support networks. This isolation contributes to the victim's increased vulnerability and difficulty in seeking help.

Financial instability and dependence can result from the abuser's control over finances. The victim may be denied access to money or resources, leaving them financially trapped and unable to leave the abusive relationship.

Disrupted sleep patterns, nightmares and flashbacks are common symptoms experienced by survivors of domestic violence. The traumatic experiences can invade their dreams and daily thoughts, leading to ongoing emotional distress.

Survivors often face challenges in forming trusting relationships and maintaining healthy ones.

In conclusion, domestic violence is a form of chronic trauma that has devastating effects on individuals and families. Recognising the dynamics of domestic violence, understanding its impact and accessing appropriate support and resources are crucial steps in the healing process. Survivors of domestic violence can find strength, resilience and empowerment as they navigate their journey towards reclaiming their lives, fostering healthy relationships and building a future free from abuse.

Remember, healing takes time. Every survivor deserves compassion, understanding and support along their path to recovery.

Childhood Abuse and Neglect

Children who experience abuse or neglect within their family environment are subject to chronic trauma. This can include physical, emotional or sexual abuse, as well as neglectful parenting or inadequate caregiving.

Childhood abuse and neglect are forms of chronic trauma that occur within the family or caregiver-child relationship. They involve the mistreatment or failure to meet a child's basic needs, resulting in significant harm to their physical, emotional or social development. Understanding the impacts of childhood abuse and neglect is essential in providing support and promoting healing for survivors.

Childhood abuse can take various forms, each with devastating consequences for the child's wellbeing. Physical abuse involves intentional actions that cause physical harm or injury to a child. It may include hitting, punching, shaking, burning or the use of objects to inflict pain. Physical abuse can result in physical injuries, such as bruises, broken bones or internal injuries, as well as long-term emotional and psychological effects.

Emotional and psychological abuse in childhood refers to the repeated and persistent mistreatment of a child that affects their emotional and psychological wellbeing. It involves behaviours and actions by caregivers or significant individuals that undermine a child's sense of self-worth, manipulates their emotions and hinders their healthy emotional development.

Types of Emotional and Psychological Abuse

Emotional and psychological abuse in childhood can take various forms.

- *Verbal abuse* involves the use of harsh, demeaning or derogatory language towards the child. Verbal abuse can include insults, belittlement, constant criticism, name-calling and yelling.

- *Rejection and neglect* can have a profound impact. It occurs when a caregiver consistently ignores or neglects a child's emotional needs, and may involve dismissing the child's emotions, withholding affection or failing to provide emotional support.

- *Gaslighting* is a manipulative tactic in which the abuser distorts the child's perception of reality. They may deny or minimise the child's experiences, manipulate their memories or make the child question their own sanity or sense of reality.

- *Emotional manipulation* involves tactics such as guilt-tripping, blame-shifting or using the child's emotions to control or manipulate their behaviour. This can create confusion, fear and a sense of powerlessness in the child.

- *Isolation* occurs when the child is intentionally kept away from social interactions and emotional support systems. The abuser may limit the child's contact with their peers, prevent them from participating in activities or intentionally isolate them from family and friends.

- *Humiliation and ridicule* involve making the child the target of jokes, sarcasm or public embarrassment. The abuser may demean the child's appearance, intelligence or abilities, leading to feelings of shame, self-doubt and low self-esteem.

Effects of Emotional and Psychological Abuse in Childhood

Emotional and psychological abuse in childhood can have significant and long-lasting effects on a child's wellbeing.

- *Low self-esteem and self-worth* is achieved through constant criticism and belittlement and can lead to feelings of worthlessness and inadequacy.

- *Emotional dysregulation* presents as the child struggling with the management and regulation of their emotions. They may exhibit difficulties in expressing emotions appropriately, have intense mood swings or struggle with emotional numbing.

- *Anxiety and depression* are common results of emotional abuse. Constant fear, uncertainty and emotional distress can significantly impact a child's mental health.

- *Social and relationship challenges* are common in children who have experienced emotional and psychological abuse. These children may find it difficult to form and maintain healthy relationships, and they may struggle with trust, intimacy and setting boundaries.

- *Cognitive and academic impairments* that influence development and performance are often seen in children who have been abused emotionally. The chronic stress and emotional turmoil may impair the child's ability to concentrate, learn and achieve their full academic potential.

Healing and Recovery

Healing from emotional and psychological abuse in childhood is a complex and ongoing process, which carry some important considerations.

- *Safety and support are paramount.* Ensuring the child's safety and providing them with a supportive and nurturing environment may involve removing the child from the abusive situation, seeking professional help and connecting with supportive individuals and resources.

- *Therapy and counselling.* Seeking professional help through trauma-informed therapy can be instrumental in the healing process. Therapists trained in working with survivors of childhood trauma can provide validation, support and guidance to navigate the complex emotions and experiences associated with abuse and neglect.

Childhood sexual abuse

Childhood sexual abuse is a deeply traumatic experience that involves the sexual exploitation or assault of a child by an adult or older person. It is a form of abuse that can have severe and long-lasting effects on the child's physical, emotional, and psychological well-being, as well as their psychological and sexual development.

Definition and Forms of Childhood Sexual Abuse

Childhood sexual abuse refers to any sexual activity involving a child that is intended for the gratification or stimulation of an adult or older person. It can take various forms, including but not limited to:

- *Contact abuse* that involves direct physical contact between the perpetrator and the child, such as fondling, penetration or oral-genital contact
- *Non-contact abuse* that does not involve direct physical contact but includes acts such as exposure to pornography, voyeurism or engaging the child in sexual conversations
- *Exploitation and grooming* involves the manipulation of a child through coercion, threats, bribery or emotional manipulation to engage in sexual activities or keep the abuse a secret.

Prevalence and Impact

Childhood sexual abuse is a widespread problem that affects individuals across different backgrounds and communities. Its impact can be profound and enduring.

- *Psychological and emotional consequences* include PTSD, depression, anxiety, self-esteem issues, shame, guilt, trust issues and difficulty forming and maintaining healthy relationships.

- *Physical health consequences*, such as chronic pain, gastrointestinal issues, sleep disturbances, substance abuse issues, eating disorders and increased risk of sexually transmitted infections (STIs) are common among survivors of childhood sexual abuse.

- *Impact on development* can include interference with cognitive development, academic performance, social skills and the development of a positive self-identity. It can also lead to precocious sexual behaviour or difficulty with sexual intimacy in adulthood.

- *The long-term effects* of childhood sexual abuse can extend into adulthood. Survivors may struggle with intimacy, sexual dysfunction, self-destructive behaviours, dissociation, revictimisation, a higher risk of mental health disorders and suicidal ideation.

Recognising and Responding to Childhood Sexual Abuse

Recognising and responding to childhood sexual abuse is crucial for the wellbeing and protection of children. There are several key steps in this process.

- *Awareness and education* about childhood sexual abuse, its signs and its consequences are essential for individuals, families, communities and professionals who interact with children.

- *Recognising the potential signs* of abuse, such as unexplained physical injuries, sudden changes in behaviour or mood, fear of certain individuals or places, sexualised behaviour or language, or withdrawal from previously enjoyed activities is crucial.

- *Creating safe environments* where children feel comfortable speaking up about abuse, can foster open communication and teach age-appropriate body boundaries and consent.

- *Reporting and seeking help* is crucial if you suspect or learn about a child experiencing sexual abuse. Reports should be made to the appropriate authorities, such as child protective services or law enforcement. Professional help, therapy and counselling can provide support for the survivor's healing process.

Healing and Support

Recovering from childhood sexual abuse is a complex and individualised journey, but there are several supportive interventions and resources available.

- *Therapeutic interventions*, such as TF-CBT, DBT or EMDR can help survivors process their experiences, manage symptoms and regain their sense of safety and self-worth.

- *Supportive relationships* with trusted individuals, such as friends, family members or support groups for survivors, can provide validation, empathy and a sense of community.

- *Self-care practices* that promote healing, such as mindfulness, meditation, exercise, journalling, art therapy or other hobbies, can assist in restoring a sense of control and self-nurturance.

- *Advocacy and empowerment* are paramount to recovery. Survivors can be supported to share their stories, advocate for change and engage in activities that promote resilience and empowerment, such as participating in support groups, volunteering or engaging in creative expression.

Healing from childhood sexual abuse is a personal and unique journey. It is essential to seek professional help, surround yourself with supportive individuals and prioritise self-care as you navigate the path towards healing and reclaiming your life.

Neglect

The failure of caregivers to meet a child's basic physical, emotional, educational or medical needs is neglect. This can include neglecting to provide food, shelter, supervision, love or protection. Neglect can lead to malnutrition, physical and developmental delays, impaired emotional regulation and difficulty forming healthy relationships. Childhood neglect is a form of chronic trauma that involves a persistent pattern of inattention and disregard for the child's wellbeing, and can have significant and long-lasting effects.

Types of Childhood Neglect

Childhood neglect can take various forms.

- *Physical Neglect* refers to a failure to provide for a child's basic physical needs, such as adequate food, clothing, shelter and medical care. It may also involve inadequate supervision or leaving the child in unsafe environments.

- *Emotional neglect* involves a lack of emotional responsiveness and support from caregivers. This can include ignoring a child's emotional needs, failing to provide affection or dismissing their feelings. Emotional neglect can create a sense of emptiness and a lack of attachment in the child.

- *Educational neglect* occurs when caregivers fail to ensure a child's access to education or do not provide adequate support for their educational development. This may involve chronic absenteeism, lack of educational resources or indifference towards the child's academic progress.

Effects of Childhood Neglect:

Childhood neglect can have significant and enduring effects on a child's development and well-being.

- *Emotional and psychological impacts* include struggles with low self-esteem, feelings of worthlessness and a sense of emptiness. Neglected children may also develop difficulties in regulating their emotions, forming healthy relationships and trusting others.

- *Cognitive and academic challenges* are common with neglected children. The lack of intellectual stimulation, educational support and consistent guidance can result in learning difficulties, poor school performance and delays in cognitive and language development.

- *Social and interpersonal difficulties* arise when neglected children experience challenges in forming and maintaining relationships. They may struggle with social skills, have difficulty establishing boundaries and exhibit a lack of empathy or understanding of the emotions of others.

- *Physical health consequences,* brought on by a lack of proper nutrition, medical care and hygiene, can lead to malnutrition, developmental delays, increased susceptibility to illness and impaired physical growth.

- *Long-term effects* of childhood neglect can extend into adulthood. Neglected individuals may experience difficulty forming healthy attachments, establishing stable employment and maintaining healthy relationships. They may also be at increased risk of mental health disorders, substance abuse and involvement in abusive relationships.

Healing and Recovery

Healing from childhood neglect is a complex and ongoing process, but it is possible to overcome the effects and build a fulfilling life.

- *Therapeutic Interventions* conducted by a mental health professional who specialises in trauma and neglect can provide essential support. Therapists can help individuals process their childhood experiences, develop coping strategies and work towards healing and self-compassion.

- *Building supportive relationships* is crucial to the healing process. Connecting with trusted friends, mentors or support groups can provide validation, empathy and a sense of belonging.

- *Self-care and self-nurturing* is essential and should be prioritised. This may involve engaging in activities that bring joy, practising self-compassion, setting healthy boundaries and focusing on personal growth and self-discovery.

- *Education and skill development* can help neglected individuals build a foundation for success and independence. This may involve pursuing formal education or vocational training to develop skills in areas of interest.

- *Advocacy and support services* can provide practical assistance and guidance. These resources can help navigate legal, educational or employment systems, and connect individuals with community resources tailored to their specific needs.

Childhood abuse and neglect can have profound and lasting effects on a child's overall wellbeing. Survivors of childhood abuse and neglect often experience a range of emotional and psychological difficulties. These can include depression, anxiety, PTSD, low self-esteem, difficulty in trusting others, self-destructive behaviours and a higher risk of developing mental health disorders later in life.

Children who experience abuse and neglect may face cognitive and developmental delays. They may have difficulties with academic performance, language development, problem-solving skills and impulse control. The chronic stress and trauma experienced during childhood can disrupt healthy brain development, affecting memory, attention and learning abilities.

Childhood abuse and neglect can significantly impact a child's ability to form healthy relationships and navigate social interactions. They may struggle with establishing trust, maintaining boundaries and understanding healthy relationship dynamics. Survivors may also be at higher risk of engaging in substance abuse, risky behaviours or experiencing further victimisation in adulthood.

Furthermore, childhood trauma can have physical health consequences that extend into adulthood. Survivors may experience higher rates of chronic health conditions, such as cardiovascular disease, obesity, autoimmune disorders and impaired immune functioning. The physiological effects of chronic stress can increase the risk of physical ailments throughout life.

Healing from childhood abuse and neglect is a complex and individualised journey, but it is possible with support and intervention. Creating a safe and stable environment is paramount for survivors, and seeking professional help through trauma-informed therapy can be instrumental in the healing process. Engaging in self-care practices, building supportive relationships and educating oneself about the impacts of childhood trauma can also aid in the healing journey.

Every survivor's path to healing is unique, and recovery is possible with time, patience and support. With appropriate interventions and support, survivors of childhood abuse and neglect can reclaim their lives, cultivate resilience and build a future free from the constraints of their past trauma.

To sum up, childhood abuse and neglect are devastating forms of chronic trauma that can have profound and lasting impacts on survivors.

Understanding the types of abuse and neglect, as well as their effects, is crucial in providing support and promoting healing. With appropriate interventions, therapy, support networks and self-care practices, survivors can embark on a journey of healing, reclaim their lives and cultivate a future free from the constraints of their past trauma. Remember, every survivor's path to healing is unique and recovery is possible with time, patience and support.

War and Political Conflict: The Impact of Prolonged Trauma

War and political conflict are harrowing experiences that disrupt the lives of individuals and communities on a massive scale. These prolonged periods of violence, upheaval and uncertainty create a pervasive environment of trauma, affecting not only the physical wellbeing of individuals but also their emotional, psychological and social dimensions. This section explores the nature of war and political conflict, their traumatic effects and the pathways to healing and resilience.

Understanding War and Political Conflict

War and political conflict encompass a broad range of situations, from armed conflicts between nations to internal conflicts within a country. They are often driven by political, ideological, ethnic or territorial disputes, resulting in widespread violence, destruction and loss of life.

- *Causes and Triggers*

Wars and political conflicts can arise from various factors, including territorial disputes, ethnic tensions, ideological differences, economic inequality and power struggles. Understanding the underlying cause is crucial to grasp the complexity of these situations.

- *Impact on Communities*

Entire communities are affected by war and political conflict, with consequences ranging from displacement and forced migration to the destruction of infrastructure, institutions and social fabric. The loss of livelihoods, access to basic services and disruption of social support systems further exacerbate the trauma experienced by individuals.

- *Historical Context*

Examining the historical context of conflicts provides insights into the cyclical nature of violence and the intergenerational transmission of trauma. Historical trauma refers to the cumulative emotional and psychological wounds passed down through generations affected by war and political conflict.

Traumatic Effects of War and Political Conflict

War and political conflict leave deep scars on individuals, families and communities. The traumatic effects extend beyond the duration of the conflict, impacting long-term wellbeing. There are some common traumatic effects.

- *Post-Traumatic Stress Disorder (PTSD)* is a prevalent psychological disorder among individuals exposed to war and political conflict. It is characterised by intrusive memories, nightmares, hypervigilance, emotional numbness and avoidance of triggers associated with the traumatic experiences. PTSD can significantly impair daily functioning and quality of life.

- *Psychological distress* extends beyond PTSD with individuals affected by war and political conflict often experiencing various forms of psychological distress. These forms can include depression, anxiety, panic attacks, survivor guilt, feelings of helplessness or hopelessness and difficulty regulating emotions.

- *Physical injuries and disabilities* are a physical toll of war and political conflict and affect combatants and civilians alike. These injuries range from gunshot wounds and amputations to traumatic brain injuries, burns and other debilitating conditions. Physical disabilities resulting from conflict can have long-term implications for an individual's functioning and well-being.

- *Displacement and refugees* are common during times of war and political conflict, where people are often forced to flee their homes. Displaced individuals and refugees face numerous challenges, including limited access to healthcare, education, employment and adequate shelter.

The experience of displacement adds another layer of trauma, often compounded by ongoing discrimination and marginalization.

- *Loss and grief* is a common consequence of war and political conflict. The grief and mourning process for the loss of loved ones, homes and livelihoods can be prolonged and complicated, leaving individuals with profound emotional pain and a sense of emptiness.

Pathways to Healing and Resilience

Although the effects of war and political conflict are devastating, healing and resilience are possible, with various approaches and interventions available to support individuals and communities on their journey towards recovery.

- *Access to mental health services* that are sensitive to cultural context and trauma-informed, is essential for addressing the psychological impact of war and political conflict. Such services may include therapy, counselling and psychiatric support.

- *Community-based support* is vital for post-conflict healing. Building community support networks and strengthening social cohesion through community-led initiatives can promote solidarity, social reintegration and collective healing processes.

- *Transitional justice* can contribute to healing and reconciliation. This includes processes such as truth commissions, reparations for victims and holding accountable those responsible for war crimes and human rights abuses.

- *Rebuilding infrastructure and institutions* is crucial for restoring normalcy and enabling communities to recover. This rebuilding may include restoring healthcare systems, educational institutions and economic structures, and are important to provide a sense of stability and hope for the future.

- *Addressing socioeconomic inequalities* is crucial for long-term peacebuilding and preventing the recurrence of violence as it is inequality that often contributes to the persistence of conflict. Efforts should focus on poverty reduction, equitable resource distribution and inclusive governance.

War and political conflict leave a profound and lasting impact on individuals and communities. Acknowledging the traumatic effects of such experiences is essential for promoting healing and resilience. By providing access to mental health services, fostering community-based support, pursuing transitional justice, rebuilding infrastructure and addressing socioeconomic inequalities, individuals and communities affected by war and political conflict can embark on a path towards healing and rebuilding their lives. Ultimately, the pursuit of peace, justice and equality is fundamental to preventing the cycle of trauma and creating a more peaceful world.

Effects of Chronic Trauma

Ongoing exposure to traumatic events and environments can have profound effects on individuals with chronic trauma.

- *Emotional and Psychological Impact*

Chronic trauma can lead to a range of emotional and psychological difficulties. These may include persistent anxiety, depression, feelings of helplessness or hopelessness, low self-esteem, difficulties in regulating emotions and a heightened sense of fear and vigilance.

- *Interpersonal Challenges*

Chronic trauma can strain relationships and interpersonal connections. Individuals who have experienced chronic trauma may struggle with trust, intimacy and forming healthy attachments. They may have difficulties expressing emotions, establishing boundaries and maintaining stable relationships.

- *Physical Health Consequences*

The impact of chronic trauma is not limited to psychological wellbeing; it can also affect physical health. Individuals may experience chronic pain, sleep disturbances, gastrointestinal issues, headaches and a weakened immune system.

- *Developmental Impacts*

When chronic trauma occurs during childhood, it can significantly impact a child's development. Children who experience ongoing trauma may have delays in cognitive, emotional and social development. They may also struggle with self-regulation, academic performance and building a sense of identity and self-worth.

Coping and Healing Strategies

While chronic trauma can have long-lasting effects, healing and recovery are possible through strategies that support individuals to cope with and heal from chronic trauma.

- *Seek Professional Help*

A qualified trauma therapist can provide valuable support and guidance. Therapists trained in trauma-focused approaches, such as CBT, DBT or EMDR, can assist individuals in processing their experiences and developing coping skills.

- *Build Supportive Relationships*

Cultivating healthy and supportive relationships is crucial in the healing process. Connecting with trusted friends, family members or support groups can provide validation, empathy and a sense of belonging.

- *Practice Self-care*

Prioritising self-care activities that promote relaxation, stress reduction and overall wellbeing can be beneficial. Engaging in activities, such as exercise, mindfulness, meditation, creative outlets and self-compassion exercises, can help individuals regain a sense of control and self-nurturance.

- *Develop Coping Strategies*

Learning effective coping strategies can assist in managing the challenges associated with chronic trauma. These may include grounding techniques, deep-breathing exercises, journalling, engaging in hobbies and seeking healthy outlets for emotions.

- *Establish Safety and Boundaries*

Creating a safe environment and setting clear boundaries are crucial in healing from chronic trauma. This may involve implementing safety plans, asserting boundaries in relationships and avoiding triggers or situations that may retraumatise.

- *Explore Healing Modalities*

Various complementary approaches can supplement traditional therapy in the healing journey. These may include art therapy, yoga, massage, acupuncture and other body-centred therapies. These modalities can help individuals reconnect with their bodies and release stored trauma.

Chronic trauma is a prolonged and ongoing experience of trauma that can deeply impact the lives of individuals. Understanding the nature of chronic trauma and its effects is essential in providing support and fostering healing. By seeking professional help, building supportive relationships, practising self-care, developing coping strategies and exploring healing modalities, individuals can embark on a path towards recovery, resilience and reclaiming their lives after chronic trauma. Healing is a unique and personal journey, and each step forward is a testament to your strength and resilience.

Complex Trauma

Complex trauma is a specific type of trauma that occurs during childhood and involves prolonged exposure to multiple traumatic events, often within the context of interpersonal relationships. It encompasses experiences such as chronic abuse, neglect or living in chronically unstable or unsafe environments. Complex trauma can have long-lasting and pervasive effects on an individual's development, shaping their beliefs, emotions and relationships throughout their lives.

Complex trauma differs from single-incident trauma or acute trauma in several key ways. While acute trauma typically involves a single traumatic event with a defined beginning and end, complex trauma is characterised by ongoing and chronic exposure to trauma. The repeated and prolonged nature of complex trauma increases the cumulative impact on the individual, making it more challenging to recover and heal.

One defining feature of complex trauma is that it often occurs within the context of close relationships, such as with caregivers or family members. These relationships, which should ideally provide safety, nurturing and support, instead become a source of fear, pain and betrayal. For example, a child subjected to chronic physical or sexual abuse by a caregiver may develop a distorted view of relationships, trust and their self-worth.

Complex trauma can disrupt multiple aspects of a child's development, including their cognitive, emotional, social and physiological functioning. The developing brain of a child is highly vulnerable and adaptable, and exposure to ongoing trauma during critical periods of brain development can have lasting effects.

Cognitive functioning is often impacted by complex trauma. The ability to concentrate, process information and learn effectively may be compromised, leading to difficulties in academic settings. Children who experience complex trauma may also have challenges with problem-solving, memory and executive functioning skills.

Emotionally, complex trauma can lead to a range of intense and conflicting emotions. These can include fear, sadness, anger, shame, guilt and confusion. Due to the chronic and unpredictable nature of the trauma, children may experience heightened emotional dysregulation, with difficulty in managing and expressing their emotions appropriately. This emotional dysregulation can persist into adulthood, impacting relationships and overall wellbeing.

Socially, complex trauma can result in difficulties in forming and maintaining healthy relationships. Trust, which is essential for building secure attachments, may be severely compromised. Individuals who have experienced complex trauma may struggle with intimacy, vulnerability and establishing healthy boundaries. They may also exhibit patterns of avoidance or disorganised attachment styles.

Physiologically, complex trauma can disrupt the stress response system, leading to ongoing hypervigilance and heightened arousal. This can manifest as sleep disturbances, chronic pain, gastrointestinal issues and an increased risk for various physical health problems. The constant state of alertness and vigilance can perpetuate a sense of danger and prevent the individual from experiencing a genuine sense of safety.

Healing from complex trauma requires a comprehensive and multidimensional approach. It often involves therapeutic interventions that address the cognitive, emotional, social and physiological aspects of the individual's experience. Trauma-focused therapies, such as TF-CBT or EMDR, can be particularly effective in helping individuals process and integrate their traumatic experiences.

In addition to therapy, creating safe and supportive environments is crucial for individuals healing from complex trauma. This includes fostering relationships with caring and reliable individuals, accessing support groups or peer support, and building a network of professionals who understand trauma and its effects.

It is important to remember that healing from complex trauma is a journey that takes time, patience and dedication. It involves unravelling deep-seated beliefs, rewiring neural pathways and cultivating resilience. With the right support and resources, individuals can gradually reclaim their lives, rebuild healthy relationships and develop a sense of empowerment and self-worth.

Complex trauma is a distinct form of trauma that occurs during childhood and involves ongoing exposure to multiple traumatic events, often within the context of interpersonal relationships. It has profound and pervasive effects on an individual's development and functioning. Healing from complex trauma requires a comprehensive approach that addresses the cognitive, emotional, social, and physiological aspects of the individual's experience. With appropriate support and therapeutic interventions, individuals can work towards healing, resilience and reclaiming their lives.

1.3 The Impact of Trauma on the Mind and Body

Trauma has a profound impact on both the mind and body of individuals. It disrupts the delicate balance of psychological and physiological functioning, leaving lasting imprints on various aspects of a person's wellbeing. In this section, we will explore the psychological and physiological effects of trauma, highlighting how it can shape an individual's thoughts, emotions, behaviours and physical health.

Psychological Impact

Trauma can have far-reaching psychological effects on individuals. It disrupts their sense of safety, control and trust, leading to a range of emotional and cognitive responses.

- *Post-Traumatic Stress Disorder (PTSD)*

PTSD is a common psychological disorder that can develop after experiencing or witnessing a traumatic event. It is characterised by a range of symptoms that persist beyond the immediate aftermath of the trauma. Symptoms can be grouped into four main clusters.

Intrusive symptoms include intrusive thoughts, memories or nightmares related to the traumatic event. Individuals with PTSD may also have intense emotional or physiological reactions when exposed to reminders of the trauma.

Avoidance symptoms include avoiding certain people, places or activities associated with the traumatic event and help sufferers cope with the distressing memories and reminders of the trauma. They may also try to push away thoughts or feelings related to the trauma, leading to emotional numbing.

Negative alterations in cognition and mood occur when trauma profoundly affects an individual's beliefs about themselves, others and the world. They may develop negative self-perceptions, feelings of guilt or shame, and a distorted view of trust and safety. There may also be persistent negative emotions, such as fear, anger and sadness, or a diminished interest in previously enjoyed activities.

Hyperarousal symptoms indicate a heightened state of physiological and psychological arousal. Individuals with PTSD may be easily startled, have difficulty concentrating or sleeping, exhibit irritability or outbursts of anger, and display hypervigilance or an exaggerated startle response. They may constantly feel on guard, as if danger is always present.

- *Anxiety and Panic Disorders*

Trauma can trigger chronic and debilitating anxiety, leading to the development of anxiety disorders. Generalised anxiety disorder involves excessive worry and apprehension about various aspects of life, and specific phobias may arise from associations with the traumatic event. Panic disorder is characterised by recurring panic attacks, which are sudden episodes of intense fear or discomfort accompanied by physical symptoms, such as heart palpitations, shortness of breath and a feeling of impending doom.

- *Depression*

Trauma increases the risk of developing depression. Individuals may experience persistent feelings of sadness, emptiness or hopelessness. They may lose interest in activities they once enjoyed and struggle with low energy levels, changes in appetite and sleep patterns, difficulty concentrating and feelings of worthlessness or guilt. Suicidal thoughts may also be present in severe cases.

- *Dissociation*

Dissociation is a defence mechanism that can occur in response to trauma. It involves a disconnection from one's thoughts, feelings, memories or sense of identity. Dissociative experiences can range from mild detachment or spacing out to more severe forms of dissociative disorders, such as dissociative amnesia, dissociative identity disorder (previously known as multiple-personality disorder), or depersonalisation/derealisation disorder. These experiences serve as a way to temporarily escape the overwhelming emotions and sensations associated with trauma.

- *Self-Esteem and Identity Issues*

Trauma can significantly impact an individual's self-esteem and sense of identity. Survivors may blame themselves for the traumatic event or internalise negative beliefs about their worth or capabilities. They may struggle with feelings of shame, guilt or self-blame. This can lead to difficulties in forming healthy relationships, setting boundaries and experiencing a sense of self-worth and empowerment.

It is important to note that the psychological impact of trauma varies from person to person. Some individuals may experience these symptoms immediately after the trauma, while others may develop them weeks, months or even years later. The severity and duration of symptoms can also vary, with some individuals experiencing chronic impairment while others may exhibit more resilient responses. Professional support and trauma-focused therapy can be instrumental in helping individuals navigate and heal from these psychological challenges.

Physiological Impact

Trauma not only affects the mind but also has significant physiological consequences. The body's stress response system becomes dysregulated, leading to a wide range of physiological symptoms.

- *Dysregulation of the Autonomic Nervous System (ANS)*

The autonomic nervous system (ANS) plays a crucial role in regulating the body's involuntary functions, including heart rate, blood pressure, digestion and respiratory rate. In individuals who have experienced trauma, the ANS can become dysregulated, leading to irregularities in these physiological processes. For example, trauma can result in an overactive sympathetic nervous system, which is responsible for the 'fight-or-flight' response that can cause heightened heart rate and blood pressure. Conversely, the parasympathetic nervous system, responsible for the body's relaxation response, may be underactive, leading to difficulties in calming down and experiencing a sense of safety.

- *Altered Neurotransmitter Levels*

Trauma can affect the levels and functioning of neurotransmitters, which are chemical messengers that facilitate communication between nerve cells in the brain. Imbalances in neurotransmitters, such as serotonin, dopamine and norepinephrine, can occur as a result of trauma. These imbalances can contribute to symptoms including mood disturbances, anxiety and difficulties with emotional regulation.

- *Impaired HPA Axis Functioning*

The hypothalamic-pituitary-adrenal (HPA) axis is a critical component of the body's stress response system. Trauma can disrupt the functioning of the HPA axis, leading to abnormal cortisol regulation. Cortisol is a stress hormone released by the adrenal glands in response to stressors. In individuals who have experienced trauma, cortisol levels may be dysregulated, with some individuals exhibiting elevated cortisol levels and others showing blunted cortisol responses. These disruptions in cortisol regulation can have wide-ranging effects on various bodily systems, including immune function, metabolism and inflammation.

- *Impact on Brain Structures and Neuroplasticity*

Trauma can affect the structure and functioning of the brain. Chronic exposure to stress and trauma can result in alterations in the size and connectivity of brain regions involved in emotion regulation, memory processing and stress response. The amygdala, which plays a key role in processing emotions and detecting threats, may become hyperactive, leading to heightened emotional reactivity. Conversely, the prefrontal cortex, responsible for executive functions such as decision-making and impulse control, may show reduced activation and connectivity, impairing these crucial cognitive processes. Neuroplasticity, the brain's ability to adapt and rewire itself, is also affected by trauma. Trauma can impact the brain's ability to form new neural connections and modify existing ones, potentially hindering the individual's ability to recover and heal.

- *Impact on the Endocrine System*

The endocrine system, which includes glands such as the thyroid, adrenal glands and reproductive organs, can be affected by trauma. Chronic stress and trauma can disrupt the balance of hormones in the body, leading to dysregulation of the menstrual cycle, decreased libido and other reproductive health issues. Trauma can also contribute to thyroid imbalances, leading to symptoms such as fatigue, weight changes and mood disturbances.

Understanding the physiological impact of trauma is essential in providing appropriate support and interventions for individuals who have experienced trauma. By recognising the interconnectedness of the mind and body, healthcare professionals can implement comprehensive approaches that address both the psychological and physiological aspects of trauma. This can include trauma-informed therapies, stress reduction techniques, physical activity and self-care practices that promote healing and restoration of physiological wellbeing.

Challenges are
opportunities for
growth. I embrace
them with an
open heart and a
calm mind

Chapter Two

Recognising the Signs and Symptoms

Trauma can have a profound impact on individuals, but its effects are not always immediately recognisable. In Chapter 2, we will explore the signs and symptoms of trauma, shedding light on how trauma can manifest in various aspects of a person's life. By increasing our understanding of these signs, we can better recognise when someone may be experiencing the effects of trauma and offer them appropriate support and resources.

2.1 Emotional Signs and Symptoms

Trauma can have a profound impact on an individual's emotional wellbeing. The emotional signs and symptoms of trauma may vary from person to person, but they often reflect the deep psychological distress caused by the traumatic experience. Recognising these signs can help us better understand and support individuals who have experienced trauma. This section will outline some of the key emotional signs and symptoms commonly associated with trauma.

Intense Anxiety and Fear

Trauma can lead to heightened levels of anxiety and fear. Individuals may experience a pervasive sense of unease and be constantly on guard, anticipating potential threats. This heightened state of anxiety can manifest as excessive worry, restlessness and a constant feeling of being 'on edge'. Individuals may also develop specific phobias or irrational fears related to their traumatic experiences. Intense anxiety and fear are common emotional signs and symptoms of trauma.

Trauma can evoke intense feelings of anxiety and fear in individuals, particularly when it involves betrayal. Betrayal can occur in various relationships, such as a close friend breaking confidentiality, a romantic partner being unfaithful or a trusted colleague undermining someone's work. The breach of trust and violation of expectations can deeply affect a person's sense of safety and security.

Case Example: Betrayal in a Romantic Relationship

Emily had been in a committed relationship with her partner Alex for several years. They shared a deep bond and Emily trusted Alex implicitly. When she discovered Alex had been having an affair behind her back for the past six months, the revelation shattered Emily's trust and left her feeling betrayed.

In the aftermath of the betrayal, Emily began experiencing intense anxiety and fear. She constantly questioned her judgement, wondering how she could have missed the signs of the affair. She found herself second-guessing her perceptions and grew hypervigilant, scanning for potential signs of further betrayal in their interactions.

The anxiety and fear Emily felt were not limited to her relationship with Alex. She found it challenging to trust others, including close friends and family. She felt vulnerable and feared that others might also betray hery. This pervasive fear began to impact Emily's ability to form new relationships or open up emotionally to others.

Additionally, Emily developed specific triggers associated with the betrayal. For example, when she encountered reminders of the affair, such as a particular song they used to enjoy together or a location they frequented, she experienced intense anxiety and intrusive thoughts about the betrayal. These triggers often resulted in heightened physiological arousal, including increased heart rate, rapid breathing and a sense of impending doom.

The intense anxiety and fear Emily experienced were not solely limited to the immediate aftermath of the betrayal. They persisted as she struggled to rebuild trust, heal from the emotional wounds and navigate the complexities of forgiveness and moving forward in the relationship.

In this example, the experience of intense anxiety and fear resulting from the betrayal highlights the profound impact trauma can have on an individual's emotional wellbeing. Emily's feelings of anxiety and fear were rooted in the breach of trust and the profound sense of vulnerability that the betrayal engendered. It is essential to acknowledge these emotional responses as they provide individuals like Emily with the support, understanding and resources necessary for healing and recovery.

Understanding the specific emotional reactions individuals may have in response to betrayal helps us to be more sensitive in our interactions. By creating a safe and non-judgemental space for individuals to express their emotions, process their experiences and rebuild trust, we can play a supportive role in their journey of healing.

Overwhelming Sadness and Depression

Trauma often brings about profound feelings of sadness and depression. Individuals may experience a deep sense of despair and hopelessness, possibly losing interest in activities they once enjoyed. Some people may struggle to find pleasure in life and have difficulty envisioning a positive future. It is important to note that trauma-related depression can be distinct from other forms of depression and may require specialised therapeutic approaches.

Case Example: Betrayal, sadness and depression

Betrayal in a close relationship, such as the discovery of infidelity, can trigger profound feelings of sadness and lead to a state of depression in the betrayed individual. The emotional impact of the betrayal can be overwhelming and may persist for an extended period.

After discovering Alex's affair, Emily was engulfed by a profound sense of sadness that seemed to permeate every aspect of her life. She found herself crying frequently, often unable to pinpoint a specific trigger for her tears. The emotional pain felt overwhelming, and Emily found it difficult to find enjoyment or pleasure in activities that she once found fulfilling.

As time went on, Emily's sadness intensified and began to take on the characteristics of depression. She felt a pervasive sense of hopelessness. Activities she once engaged in with enthusiasm now felt meaningless and empty. She withdrew from social interactions, finding it challenging to muster the energy or motivation to engage with others. Even daily tasks became burdensome, and she struggled to find the motivation to care for herself.

Sleep disturbances became another hallmark of Emily's depression. She found it increasingly difficult to fall asleep, often lying awake for hours with racing thoughts. When she did manage to fall asleep, her sleep was disrupted by vivid and distressing dreams related to the betrayal. Consequently, she woke up exhausted and lacked the energy to face the day.

The overwhelming sadness and depression also impacted Emily's self-esteem and self-worth. She began to question her value and blamed herself for the betrayal. She constantly replayed the events in her mind, searching for flaws or signs that she may have contributed to the betrayal. This self-blame only intensified her feelings of sadness and further eroded her sense of self.

It is important to note that overwhelming sadness and depression resulting from betrayal can be distinct from other forms of depression. The underlying cause and context of the betrayal can significantly influence the individual's emotional experience. In Emily's case, the betrayal shook the foundation of her relationship and shattered her trust, leading to a profound and prolonged period of sadness and depression.

Recognising the depth of the sadness and depression that individuals like Emily experience is crucial in providing appropriate support. Encouraging open and compassionate communication, validating their emotions, and connecting them with professional help, such as therapy, can be instrumental in their healing journey. Additionally, fostering a safe and supportive environment where they feel heard, understood and valued can aid in their recovery from the emotional impact of the betrayal.

Intrusive Memories and Flashbacks

Traumatic experiences, such as the discovery of betrayal, can give rise to intrusive memories and flashbacks. These involuntary and distressing recollections of the traumatic event can intrude upon an individual's thoughts and disrupt their daily life.

Case Example: The role of memory

Following the discovery of Alex's affair, Emily began to experience intrusive memories related to the betrayal. These memories would come to her unexpectedly, often triggered by reminders associated with the affair, such as certain locations, objects, or even words. For example, seeing a restaurant they used to frequent together or hearing a particular song they shared could trigger vivid recollections of the painful moments she discovered the affair.

In Emily's case, her intrusive memories were distressing and often brought forth intense emotions. She would find herself reliving the events of the betrayal as if they were happening all over again. The emotions, sensory details and physical sensations she experienced during the initial discovery of the affair would flood her consciousness, overwhelming her with a sense of helplessness and anguish.

Emily also experienced flashbacks. More immersive, flashbacks can feel as though the traumatic event is happening in the present moment. During a flashback, Emily would often lose touch with her current surroundings, becoming fully immersed in the traumatic memory. A rapid heartbeat, shallow breathing and a sense of panic or distress were common as the emotions and sensations associated with the betrayal overwhelmed her.

Emily's daily life was not only disrupted but the intrusive memories and flashbacks also contributed to heightened anxiety and hypervigilance. She found herself constantly on edge, anticipating triggers and becoming hyper-aware of her surroundings as she tried to avoid situations that could elicit pain in this way.

It is important to note that intrusive memories and flashbacks are involuntary and can be extremely distressing for individuals who have experienced trauma as they are disruptive and can significantly impact their quality of life. Understanding the nature of intrusive memories and flashbacks can help us offer support and empathy to individuals like Emily.

Supportive interventions for managing intrusive memories and flashbacks may include grounding techniques, such as deep breathing exercises, mindfulness practices or focusing on sensory experiences, and can bring individuals back to the present moment. Seeking professional help from a therapist trained in trauma-focused therapies, such as Eye Movement Desensitization and Reprocessing (EMDR) or Cognitive-Behavioural Therapy (CBT), can also be beneficial in processing and reducing the impact of intrusive memories and flashbacks.

Creating a safe and non-judgemental environment, where individuals feel comfortable discussing their experiences and offering validation for their emotions, can contribute to healing and recovery. By acknowledging the distress caused by intrusive memories and flashbacks, we can support individuals like Emily to find effective coping strategies and gradually reclaim control over their lives.

Emotional Numbing and Detachment

Trauma, such as the discovery of betrayal, can lead to emotional numbing and detachment as a coping mechanism. This defensive response helps individuals protect themselves from overwhelming emotions and can manifest in various ways.

Case Example: Connection and detachment

Following the betrayal, Emily found it increasingly challenging to connect with her own emotions and the emotions of others; in other words, she was experiencing a sense of emotional numbing. It was as if a protective shield had formed around her, creating a barrier between herself and the world. She noticed that the once vibrant range of her emotions had become muted, leaving her emotionally detached.

One manifestation of emotional numbing was the difficulty Emily faced in trying to express her feelings. She struggled to articulate her emotions and found herself detached, even when situations called for an emotional response. It became challenging for her to access and convey her true emotions, leading to disconnection from herself and others.

Emily also experienced detachment in her interpersonal relationships. She found it challenging to trust others and establish deep emotional connections.

The betrayal had eroded her faith in others, causing her to keep people at a distance to protect herself from potential pain and betrayal. Emily withdrew from social interactions and became guarded in her interactions, fearing that any vulnerability could lead to further hurt.

This emotional detachment not only impacted her relationships but also her ability to experience joy and pleasure. Activities that once brought her happiness now felt distant and unfulfilling. The emotional colour that infused her life seemed to have faded, leaving her in a state of emotional emptiness.

It is important to understand that emotional numbing and detachment are not conscious choices but protective responses to overwhelming emotions and the fear of being hurt again. While they serve as coping mechanisms in the short term, over time, they can hinder healing and the restoration of emotional wellbeing.

Supportive interventions for individuals experiencing emotional numbing and detachment may involve creating a safe and non-judgemental space where they can explore their emotions at their own pace. Encouraging self-compassion and self-care can also help individuals reconnect with their emotions and gradually open themselves up to emotional experiences.

Professional support from a therapist can be beneficial in navigating the complex emotions associated with betrayal and trauma. Therapies such as CBT, Dialectical Behaviour Therapy (DBT) or other trauma-focused therapies can help individuals process their emotions, challenge negative beliefs and develop healthier coping mechanisms.

By fostering an environment of understanding, patience and support, we can help individuals like Emily on their journey towards healing. Recognising and validating their experience of emotional numbing and detachment can contribute to their ability to reconnect with their emotions, rebuild trust and establish meaningful connections with others.

Anger and Irritability

Traumatic experiences, such as betrayal, can trigger intense feelings of anger and irritability in individuals. The sense of injustice and violation that accompany betrayal can ignite a range of angry emotions.

Case Example: The deep well of anger

Following the discovery of Alex's affair, Emily experienced a surge of anger. The profound sense of betrayal and violation of trust stirred within her a deep well of anger. This anger was directed at both Alex and herself. She was furious with Alex for the breach of their commitment and the pain he caused. At the same time, she harboured self-directed anger for not recognising the signs earlier or for potentially contributing to the betrayal in some way.

Emily's anger manifested in various ways. She often found herself feeling irritable and easily provoked by minor annoyances. Small inconveniences she might have brushed off before now magnified her anger. She became short-tempered and had difficulty controlling her outbursts of frustration. These episodes of anger and irritability not only strained her relationships with others but also added to her feelings of guilt and shame.

Furthermore, the anger Emily experienced was not limited to specific moments of frustration or irritation. It lingered beneath the surface, simmering as a constant undercurrent in her interactions and thoughts. She developed a deep resentment towards Alex, which coloured her perception of him and their relationship. This anger sometimes spilled over into her interactions with others, as she struggled to trust and connect with people, fearing that they too might betray her.

It is important to note that anger, when experienced in response to betrayal, is a natural and valid emotional response. It can serve as a protective mechanism, asserting boundaries and signalling a need for justice and accountability. However, unresolved anger can hinder the healing process and contribute to further distress.

Supportive interventions for individuals struggling with anger and irritability may involve providing them with a safe space to express and explore their anger constructively. Encouraging healthy outlets for anger, such as engaging in physical activity, writing in a journal or seeking support from a therapist, can help individuals productively process their emotions.

Therapeutic approaches like CBT or anger management techniques can assist individuals in understanding the underlying causes of their anger, challenging distorted thinking patterns and developing healthier coping strategies.

Creating an environment of empathy and understanding, where individuals like Emily feel validated in their emotions, can contribute to their healing and provide a framework for addressing and transforming their anger. Through self-reflection, emotional expression, and targeted interventions, individuals can navigate through their anger and work towards resolution and growth.

Overwhelming Guilt and Shame

Discovering betrayal in a close relationship can often lead to overwhelming feelings of guilt and shame in the betrayed individual. These emotions can stem from various sources, including self-blame, questioning one's worth, or internalising the betrayal as a reflection of personal failures.

Case Example: Questioning yourself

Upon learning about Alex's affair, Emily was consumed by a profound sense of guilt. She began to question herself and her actions leading up to the betrayal. Thoughts such as, "If only I had been more attentive," or "Maybe I'm not lovable enough," plagued her mind. She blamed herself for not recognising the signs earlier or for potentially contributing to the relationship breakdown. This self-blame intensified her guilt and further eroded her self-esteem.

Additionally, Emily experienced a deep sense of shame. She felt that the betrayal reflected on her as a person; as if she had failed. Shame can be a powerful and pervasive emotion, often leading individuals to believe they are fundamentally flawed or unworthy of love and respect. Emily internalised the betrayal as a reflection of her worthiness, thus reinforcing her feelings of shame.

The overwhelming guilt and shame affected various aspects of Emily's life. She withdrew from social interactions, isolating herself from friends and loved ones out of fear of judgement and exposure. The shame she felt prevented her from seeking support or sharing her experience, as she believed that others would view her as weak or inadequate.

Furthermore, guilt and shame influenced Emily's self-perception. She struggled with feelings of inadequacy and questioned her ability to trust and form meaningful connections in the future. The weight of guilt and shame overshadowed her sense of self-worth, leaving her feeling trapped in a cycle of negative self-perception.

It is crucial to recognise that overwhelming guilt and shame in response to betrayal are common and often unwarranted. It is important to remind individuals like Emily that they are not to blame for someone else's choices or actions. Encouraging self-compassion and self-forgiveness can help alleviate the burden of guilt and shame.

Supportive interventions for individuals grappling with overwhelming guilt and shame may involve providing a safe and non-judgemental space for them to explore and process their emotions. Guiding them toward self-reflection and challenging negative self-perceptions can help them reframe their experiences and cultivate a more compassionate understanding of themselves.

Therapeutic approaches, such as CBT, Acceptance and Commitment Therapy (ACT) or self-compassion exercises, can aid individuals to address guilt and shame, foster self-forgiveness and rebuild their self-esteem.

By fostering an environment of empathy and understanding, we can support individuals like Emily in recognising that the weight of guilt and shame does not define their worth. Offering reassurance, validation and assistance to reframe their experiences can contribute to healing and enable individuals to rebuild their sense of self.

Emotional Dysregulation

Trauma, such as the discovery of betrayal, can disrupt a person's emotional regulation, leading to difficulties in managing and controlling their emotions. Emotional dysregulation refers to a state where emotions become overwhelming and challenging to navigate effectively.

Case Example: Managing emotions

Following the betrayal, Emily experienced significant challenges in regulating her emotions. Her emotional landscape became tumultuous and unpredictable. She found it difficult to control the intensity and duration of her emotional reactions, often feeling overwhelmed by waves of sadness, anger, fear and despair.

One aspect of emotional dysregulation for Emily was the experience of intense mood swings. Her emotions would fluctuate rapidly, shifting from periods of deep sadness to bursts of anger or irritability. These sudden shifts made it challenging for her to maintain emotional stability, as her moods would seem to change without warning.

Additionally, Emily struggled with heightened sensitivity to emotional triggers. Even events or comments that seemed innocuous could elicit intense emotional responses. For example, a passing mention of infidelity in a movie or a couple's public display of affection could trigger a flood of emotions and intensify Emily's feelings of sadness, anger or jealousy.

Another manifestation of emotional dysregulation for Emily was the difficulty she experienced managing and expressing her emotions appropriately. She sometimes felt overwhelmed by the intensity of her emotions and found it challenging to articulate her feelings or needs effectively. This sometimes led to anger and frustration, or conversely, a complete shut-down and withdrawal from emotional expression.

Furthermore, Emily experienced difficulty in finding emotional balance and stability. Her emotions were constantly in flux, making it challenging to find a stable emotional baseline. This instability further contributed to her sense of unease and heightened distress.

It's important to note that emotional dysregulation is a common response to trauma; in this case, the betrayal. Traumatic experiences can disrupt the brain's normal emotion regulation process and amplify emotional responses.

Supportive interventions for individuals struggling with emotional dysregulation may involve teaching techniques for emotion regulation, such as deep-breathing exercises, grounding techniques or mindfulness practices. Encouraging self-care activities, such as engaging in hobbies, practising relaxation techniques or seeking professional help from a therapist trained in trauma-focused therapies, can also be beneficial.

Therapeutic approaches, including DBT or Emotion-Focused Therapy (EFT) can help individuals develop strategies for emotional regulation and cultivate a greater sense of emotional balance. These approaches focus on identifying and understanding emotions, developing healthy coping mechanisms and building emotional resilience.

Creating a supportive and non-judgemental environment where individuals in Emily's position feel safe to express and explore their emotions can contribute to their healing process. By offering empathy, validation and tools for emotional regulation, we can assist them in finding greater stability and a sense of control over their emotional experiences.

It is essential to approach individuals experiencing these emotional signs and symptoms with compassion, empathy and non-judgement. Trauma can deeply impact emotional wellbeing, and validating an individual's experiences, while providing a safe space for expression, is crucial.

In the next section, we will explore the behavioural signs and symptoms of trauma, shedding light on how trauma can influence an individual's actions and interactions with others.

2.2 Behavioural Signs and Symptoms

The effects of trauma can be observed in an individual's behaviour and daily functioning. In this section, we will continue to use the case of Emily and Alex to provide context for the discussion. There are several common behavioural signs and symptoms associated with trauma.

Avoidance Behaviours

In the aftermath of trauma, such as the betrayal experienced by Emily, individuals may develop avoidance behaviours as a way to protect themselves from distressing memories, emotions or reminders of the traumatic event. Avoidance behaviours can manifest in various ways and often serve as coping mechanisms to minimise exposure to triggers associated with the trauma.

In Emily's case, after discovering Alex's affair, she began exhibiting avoidance behaviours to shield herself from the pain and reminders of the betrayal. Following are some common examples of avoidance behaviours.

- *Avoiding Certain Places*

Emily may actively avoid places that hold significant memories with Alex. For instance, she might avoid their favourite restaurant, parks they used to visit or even certain streets or neighbourhoods that trigger painful memories of their relationship.

- *Withdrawing from Social Interactions*

Emily may prefer to isolate herself rather than face the discomfort of discussing the betrayal or being around mutual friends who may remind her of the relationship. She may decline invitations to social events or cut off contact with certain individuals to minimise the chances of encountering triggers associated with her trauma.

- *Avoiding Emotional Triggers*

Emily might go to great lengths to avoid emotional triggers that remind her of the betrayal. This could include avoiding certain movies, songs or activities she once enjoyed with Alex. She may avoid conversations or topics related to infidelity, or relationships in general, to prevent stirring up painful emotions.

- *Suppressing or Avoiding Emotional Expression*

Emily may find it challenging to express her emotions openly or engage in discussions about her feelings surrounding the betrayal. She may avoid talking about her pain or may actively suppress her emotions as a way to protect herself from further distress. This can lead to emotional detachment or a reluctance to engage in deep emotional connections with others.

It is important to note that avoidance behaviours, while initially serving as a protective mechanism, can hinder the healing process. Avoiding triggers and emotions associated with trauma can prevent individuals from fully processing and integrating their experiences, potentially prolonging their distress.

Supportive interventions for individuals exhibiting avoidance behaviours may involve gently encouraging them to confront and explore their triggers and emotions at a pace that feels manageable. This can be done through therapy, where a safe and supportive environment is provided for individuals to work through their trauma-related challenges. Gradual exposure to triggers, in a controlled and supported manner, can help individuals build resilience and reduce avoidance behaviours over time.

Therapeutic approaches such as CBT or EMDR can be beneficial in addressing avoidance behaviours and facilitating the processing of traumatic experiences. These approaches can help individuals challenge their avoidance patterns, develop healthier coping strategies and gradually reintegrate aspects of their lives that they have been avoiding.

By fostering understanding, patience and empathy, we can support individuals in Emily's situation to navigate their avoidance behaviours, and help them find a balance between self-care and gradual exposure to triggers, ultimately facilitating their healing and growth.

Social Withdrawal and Isolation

Trauma can lead to individuals having difficulty trusting others, fearing being hurt again or feeling disconnected from those around them. They may withdraw from social interactions, have difficulty forming or maintaining relationships, and prefer to spend time alone.

Following a traumatic event like betrayal, individuals may experience a strong desire to withdraw from social interactions and isolate themselves from others. This behaviour serves as a way to protect themselves from potential judgement, further emotional pain, or triggers associated with the trauma. In Emily's case, the discovery of Alex's affair may have led to social withdrawal and isolation. There are several ways these behaviours may have manifested.

- *Decreased Social Engagements*

Emily may have reduced her participation in social activities, events and gatherings. She might decline invitations from friends, avoid group outings or make excuses to avoid socialising. By limiting her social engagements, Emily creates a sense of safety and minimises exposure to situations that could trigger painful emotions or reminders of her betrayed relationship.

- *Withdrawing from Mutual Friends*

Emily may choose to distance herself from the friends she shared with Alex. This withdrawal allows Emily to avoid uncomfortable conversations or reminders of the betrayal. She might hesitate to confide in these friends due to concerns about their loyalty or potential ties to Alex and even cut off contact or limit interactions with these individuals.

- *Avoiding Intimate Relationships*

Emily may find herself hesitant to pursue new romantic relationships. The fear of vulnerability and the potential for re-experiencing the pain of betrayal may cause her to put up emotional barriers or avoid getting close to others. This withdrawal serves as a protective mechanism to shield herself from potential hurt.

Self-Imposed Isolation

Emily may choose to spend an excessive amount of time alone, intentionally isolating herself from others. This isolation can provide a sense of safety and control, allowing her to process her emotions and avoid potential triggers. However, prolonged isolation can exacerbate feelings of loneliness, sadness and disconnection from the support and understanding of others.

Social withdrawal and isolation can be detrimental to an individual's wellbeing as they can contribute to feelings of loneliness, exacerbate depressive symptoms and hinder the healing process. It is important to approach individuals exhibiting these behaviours with sensitivity and support.

Supportive interventions for individuals experiencing social withdrawal and isolation may involve gently encouraging them to engage in social activities at their own pace. This could include inviting them to low-pressure social gatherings or supporting them to reconnect with trusted friends or family members. Providing a safe and non-judgemental space for them to express their emotions and concerns can also be beneficial.

Therapeutic interventions such as individual counselling or support groups can offer a supportive environment for individuals to process their experiences, share their feelings and connect with others who have gone through similar challenges. Therapies such as ACT or Interpersonal Psychotherapy (IPT) can assist individuals to rebuild social connections, improve communication skills and address any underlying issues contributing to their withdrawal.

By fostering understanding, patience and empathy, we can support individuals like Emily to navigate social withdrawal and isolation. Encouraging them to reach out for support, providing opportunities for social connection and promoting self-compassion can help facilitate their healing process and gradual integration back into social relationships.

Changes in Relationships

Trauma can significantly impact an individual's relationships. They may struggle with intimacy, have difficulty trusting others and experience challenges in establishing and maintaining healthy boundaries. The effects of trauma can strain familial relationships, friendships and romantic partnerships.

Trauma, particularly relational trauma like betrayal, can profoundly impact an individual's relationships. The dynamics and trust within existing relationships may undergo significant changes, and new challenges can arise in forming new connections. In the case of Emily and Alex, the betrayal has likely caused noticeable changes in their relationship, as well as in Emily's approach to future relationships. Following is a closer look at how these changes in relationships may manifest.

- *Trust Issues*

The betrayal experienced by Emily can result in deep-seated trust issues, not only in her relationship with Alex but also in her ability to trust others. Trust, which forms the foundation of healthy relationships, has been shattered, leading to scepticism and caution when forming new connections. Emily may find it challenging to trust the intentions of others, leading to a guarded approach in her interactions.

- *Emotional Guardedness*

As a protective response, Emily may become emotionally guarded, keeping her emotions and vulnerabilities hidden to prevent further hurt. She may erect emotional barriers as a defense mechanism, making it difficult for others to get close to her, or for her to express her true feelings. This guardedness can hinder the development of deep emotional intimacy in future relationships.

- *Fear of Intimacy*

The betrayal experienced by Emily can instill a fear of intimacy and a reluctance to open up emotionally in future relationships. She may be hesitant to invest in new relationships, fearing the potential for similar pain and betrayal. This fear can manifest as a desire to maintain distance or to keep relationships superficial to avoid vulnerability.

- *Difficulty Forming New Connections*

Following a traumatic event, individuals may find it challenging to form new connections and establish trusting relationships. Emily may struggle to initiate new relationships or may have heightened criteria for selecting potential partners. This cautious approach is an attempt to protect herself from experiencing similar pain and betrayal again.

- *Re-evaluating Existing Relationships*

The betrayal experienced by Emily may cause her to re-evaluate her existing relationships, including friendships and family connections. She may question the loyalty and trustworthiness of those around her, leading to increased scepticism and a need for reassurance. This re-evaluation can strain relationships and create an emotional distance between Emily and her support system.

Navigating these changes in relationships requires patience, understanding and supportive interventions. Emily needs to have a space to process her emotions, address her trust issues and develop healthier relationship patterns. There are a range of supportive interventions that can be helpful.

- *Individual Counselling*

Emily may benefit from individual counselling to explore her feelings, address trust issues and work through the emotional aftermath of the betrayal. A therapist can provide guidance, support and tools to help rebuild trust, manage fear of intimacy and develop healthier relationship patterns.

- *Supportive Friends and Family*

Having a supportive network of friends and family who can provide empathy, understanding and non-judgemental support is crucial. These individuals can help create a sense of safety and provide reassurance as Emily works through her trust issues and adjusts to the changes in her relationships.

- *Patience and Self-Compassion*

It is important Emily is patient with herself and practises self-compassion. Healing and rebuilding trust both take time. It is okay to set boundaries and take things at a pace that feels comfortable.

By providing a supportive and understanding environment, individuals like Emily can gradually heal from the impact of betrayal and develop healthier relationship patterns. With time, self-reflection and professional guidance, it is possible to rebuild trust, form new connections and cultivate meaningful relationships based on mutual respect and understanding.

Self-Destructive Behaviours

Some individuals who have experienced trauma may engage in self-destructive behaviours as a way to cope with their emotional pain. This can include substance abuse, self-harm or engaging in risky behaviours. These behaviours may offer temporary relief from distress but can have long-term detrimental effects on their wellbeing.

Traumatic experiences, such as betrayal, can sometimes lead individuals to engage in self-destructive behaviours as a way to cope with overwhelming emotions or to express their pain and distress. These behaviours are often maladaptive and can harm an individual's physical and emotional wellbeing. In the case of Emily, Alex's betrayal may trigger one of several self-destructive behaviours.

- *Substance Abuse*

Emily may turn to alcohol, drugs or other substances as a way to escape or numb her emotional pain. Substance abuse may temporarily provide a sense of relief or distraction, but can ultimately exacerbate emotional distress and create additional problems.

- *Self-Harm*

Emily may engage in behaviours such as cutting, burning or hitting herself, as a way to cope with emotional pain. Self-harm can serve as a maladaptive coping mechanism to release intense emotions or regain a sense of control. However, it is important to note that self-harm is not a healthy or effective way to manage emotional distress and should be addressed with professional help.

- *Reckless or Impulsive Behaviour*

Emily may engage in dangerous driving, risky sexual encounters or excessive spending as a way to seek temporary relief or a sense of control. These behaviours can put her safety and wellbeing at risk and may have long-term consequences.

- *Disordered Eating*

The betrayal experienced by Emily may trigger disordered eating behaviours, such as restrictive eating, binge eating or purging. These behaviours can be attempts to gain a sense of control over her emotions or body. Disordered eating can have significant physical and psychological health consequences and requires professional intervention.

- *Self-Isolation*

Emily may isolate herself from social support systems, denying herself the connection and support she needs to heal. This self-imposed isolation can intensify feelings of loneliness and contribute to a downward spiral of negative emotions.

It is important to approach individuals exhibiting self-destructive behaviours with compassion, understanding and professional support. Some supportive interventions that can be helpful include:

- seeking professional help from a therapist, counsellor or psychiatrist can provide the necessary guidance and support to address self-destructive behaviours. A mental health professional can help explore healthier coping strategies, manage emotions and develop resilience.

- creating a safety plan with the help of a mental health professional is important when the individual is engaging in immediate or severe self-destructive behaviours. A safety plan outlines strategies for managing intense emotions, identifying triggers and reaching out for support during crises.

- encouraging healthy coping mechanisms such as exercise, journalling, engaging in creative outlets, practising mindfulness or meditation, and seeking social support can provide alternative ways to manage emotions and express pain.

- reaching out to a support network, such as friends, family or groups provides a safe space to express emotions and the ability to access appropriate resources. Support networks offer understanding, empathy and non-judgemental support.

- engaging in psychoeducation about the consequences of self-destructive behaviours can help individuals understand the importance of seeking help and engaging in positive coping strategies. Information and resources about self-destructive behaviours, their impact and healthier alternatives can empower people to make informed choices and take steps towards recovery.

It is crucial to emphasise that professional help is essential when dealing with self-destructive behaviours. A mental health professional can tailor interventions to Emily's specific needs and provide appropriate support and guidance throughout her healing journey.

Hypervigilance and Startle Response

Trauma can heighten an individual's sense of threat and lead to hypervigilance. They may constantly scan their environment for potential dangers, have an exaggerated startle response and be easily overwhelmed by sensory stimuli.

Following a traumatic event like betrayal, hypervigilance and an exaggerated startle response are part of the body's natural defence mechanism and serve to maintain a state of constant alertness and readiness for potential threats. In the case of Emily, the betrayal by Alex may have triggered these responses, which then manifested in various ways.

- *Hypervigilance*

When hypervigilant, Emily may find herself in a state of heightened alertness and increased sensitivity to potential threats. She may be constantly scanning her environment, and anticipating potential signs of deception or betrayal from others. Emily may become excessively vigilant, constantly on guard and suspicious of the motives and intentions of those around her.

When interacting with new acquaintances, for example, Emily may be hypervigilant, paying close attention to their behaviour, words and actions, and searching for any potential signs of betrayal or untrustworthiness. This hypervigilance can be exhausting and can lead to feelings of anxiety, fear and difficulty relaxing or letting her guard down.

- *Exaggerated Startle Response*

Emily may also become easily startled or jumpy, even in response to minor stimuli. For instance, a sudden noise or an unexpected touch may trigger an intense physical and emotional reaction, causing her heart rate to increase, muscles to tense and a sense of impending danger or threat.

The heightened startle response can be a result of the heightened state of alertness and the heightened activation of the body's stress response system. It reflects an individual's increased sensitivity to potential dangers and an instinctive readiness to react and protect themselves.

It is important to understand that hypervigilance and an exaggerated startle response are natural responses to trauma. However, when they persist over time and significantly impact daily functioning, they may require intervention and support, including:

- psychoeducation to normalise Emily's experiences and alleviate some of the associated distress. Being provided with information about hypervigilance and the exaggerated startle response can help people understand they are common reactions to trauma.

- grounding techniques to help manage hypervigilance and startle responses. These techniques can involve engaging the senses to bring attention to the present moment, such as deep-breathing exercises, mindfulness practices or focusing on specific sensory experiences (e.g. feeling the texture of an object or listening to calming music). Grounding techniques also help direct attention away from perceived threats and promote a sense of safety and calm.

- relaxation and stress reduction techniques, such as progressive muscle relaxation, meditation or yoga, can help reduce overall stress levels and promote a sense of calm. They are valuable tools for managing hypervigilance and mitigating the startle response.

- Cognitive-Behavioural Therapy (CBT) can be beneficial for addressing hypervigilance and exaggerated startle responses. A therapist can help Emily identify and challenge negative or distorted thoughts that contribute to her heightened state of alertness. Through CBT, techniques can be learned to reframe thoughts, reduce anxiety and gradually re-establish safety and trust in her environment.

- Eye Movement Desensitisation and Reprocessing (EMDR) is a specialised therapeutic approach that can be effective in treating trauma-related symptoms, including hypervigilance and startle responses. This therapy involves bilateral stimulation (e.g. eye movements or tactile stimulation) while focusing on traumatic memories to facilitate their processing and desensitisation. EMDR can help reduce the intensity of these symptoms and promote healing.

By implementing these interventions and seeking professional help, Emily can gradually reduce hypervigilance and manage her exaggerated startle response, allowing her to regain a sense of safety and control in her daily life.

Changes in Sleep and Eating Patterns

Trauma can disrupt an individual's sleep and eating patterns. They may experience difficulties falling asleep, staying asleep or having restful sleep. Similarly, trauma can lead to changes in appetite, resulting in either a significant increase or decrease in food intake.

Disruption of an individual's sleep and eating patterns can affect their overall wellbeing. These changes can manifest in various ways, and in Emily's case, Alex's betrayal may have triggered alterations in her sleep and eating habits, causing changes to manifest.

- *Sleep Disturbances*

Emily may experience difficulties falling asleep, staying asleep or experiencing restful sleep. She may have intrusive thoughts, nightmares or vivid dreams related to the betrayal, which can also disrupt her sleep. Additionally, hypervigilance and heightened anxiety can keep her in a state of arousal, making it challenging to relax and fall asleep.

Conversely, some individuals may respond to trauma by sleeping excessively as a way to escape from distressing emotions or to withdraw from the overwhelming reality. This excessive sleep can be a form of avoidance or an attempt to find solace.

- *Insomnia*

Emily may develop insomnia, which is characterised by persistent difficulties falling asleep or staying asleep. Insomnia can be a result of anxiety, intrusive thoughts or hyperarousal related to the betrayal. The distressing emotions associated with the event can make it challenging for Emily to quiet her mind and find the calm necessary for restful sleep.

- *Changes in Appetite*

Following the betrayal, Emily's appetite may have been affected, leading to changes in her eating patterns. This may be a loss of appetite, resulting in weight loss and nutritional deficiencies. individuals may respond to trauma by using food as a source of comfort, leading to overeating and weight gain. Emotional eating can be a way to temporarily numb or distract from distressing emotions.

- *Disruptions in Eating Schedule*

Trauma can disrupt an individual's regular eating schedule. Emily may have irregular meal times or skip meals altogether due to heightened stress, emotional distress or preoccupation with the betrayal. In some cases, trauma can lead to disordered eating patterns, such as binge eating or restrictive eating behaviours.

It is important to approach changes in sleep and eating patterns with empathy and understanding as they are common reactions to trauma. Some supportive interventions that can be helpful include:

- establishing a sleep routine can promote better sleep hygiene. This involves going to bed and waking up at the same time each day, creating a relaxing bedtime routine, and ensuring the sleep environment is conducive to restful sleep (e.g., comfortable bedding, a dark and quiet room).

- relaxation techniques, such as deep breathing exercises, progressive muscle relaxation or guided imagery, can help Emily relax before bed and reduce anxiety and hypervigilance. These techniques can promote a sense of calm and improve sleep quality.

- Cognitive-behavioural therapy for Insomnia (CBT-I) can be beneficial. This therapeutic approach targets the underlying thoughts, emotions and behaviours that contribute to insomnia. A therapist can help Emily develop strategies to reframe negative thoughts, establish healthy sleep habits and improve sleep quality.

- balanced eating habits include consuming a nutritious diet that incorporates a variety of food groups and regular meal times. Encouraging mindful eating, where Emily pays attention to her body's hunger and fullness cues, can also be helpful and support her overall wellbeing.

- seeking professional help from a therapist or healthcare provider may be beneficial if Emily's sleep disturbances or changes in eating patterns persist and significantly impact her daily functioning. They can assess her specific needs and provide guidance, support and appropriate treatment options.

By addressing the changes in sleep and eating patterns and seeking the necessary support, Emily can work towards restoring a healthier balance in her sleep and eating habits, contributing to her overall healing and wellbeing.

Academic or Occupational Challenges

The effects of trauma can extend to an individual's academic or occupational functioning. They may have difficulty concentrating, experience memory impairments and struggle to meet academic or work-related responsibilities. Trauma-related symptoms can affect their overall productivity and success in these domains.

Traumatic experiences can significantly impact an individual's ability to function effectively in academic or occupational settings. The distress, emotional turmoil, and cognitive disruptions associated with trauma can manifest in various ways, affecting their performance and overall functioning. In the case of Emily, the betrayal may have resulted in academic or occupational challenges.

- *Concentration and Focus Difficulties*

Following the betrayal, Emily may experience difficulties concentrating and maintaining focus. Intrusive thoughts related to the event, emotional distress and a heightened state of alertness can make it challenging to direct her attention towards academic or work tasks. This may result in decreased productivity, reduced efficiency and difficulty completing assignments or tasks on time.

- *Memory Impairment*

Trauma can impact an individual's memory and cognitive functioning. Emily may struggle with memory impairment, such as difficulty recalling information, remembering details or retaining new information. This can hinder her ability to learn and perform optimally in academic or occupational settings.

- *Decreased Motivation and Engagement*

The emotional impact of betrayal can lead to decreased motivation and engagement in academic or work-related activities. Emily may find it challenging to feel enthusiastic or interested in her studies or job due to feelings of betrayal, sadness or disillusionment. This can result in reduced productivity, a decline in performance and a lack of fulfilment.

- *Interpersonal Difficulties*

The betrayal experienced by Emily can affect her interpersonal relationships in academic or occupational settings. She may struggle with trust issues, leading to difficulties forming new connections or maintaining existing ones. These challenges can result in isolation, alienation and decreased collaboration or teamwork.

Absenteeism or Presenteeism

Trauma can lead to increased absenteeism or presenteeism in academic or occupational settings. Emily may find it challenging to attend classes or work regularly due to emotional distress, physical symptoms or difficulties managing the impact of the betrayal. Alternatively, she may physically be present but struggle to perform effectively due to emotional and cognitive disruptions.

Addressing academic or occupational challenges requires understanding, support and appropriate interventions.

- Establishing supportive environments in academic or occupational settings can help alleviate some of the challenges. This can include fostering open communication, providing understanding and flexible accommodations and promoting a culture of empathy and support.

- Seeking academic or occupational support services can provide Emily with the resources and assistance she needs. This may include seeking guidance from academic advisors, career counsellors or human resource professionals who can provide tailored support based on her specific challenges and needs.

- Time management and organisational skill development can enhance Emily's ability to prioritise tasks, manage deadlines and maintain focus. This can help mitigate some of the academic or occupational challenges she may be facing.

- Cognitive-behavioural techniques, such as goal-setting, cognitive restructuring and stress management strategies, can help address academic or occupational challenges. A therapist or counsellor can guide Emily in developing these techniques to manage negative thoughts, enhance motivation and improve overall performance.

- Self-care and stress management can have a positive impact on academic or occupational functioning. Engaging in activities that promote relaxation, maintaining a healthy work-life balance and seeking emotional support can contribute to wellbeing and resilience in these settings.

Remember, each individual's experience and challenges may vary. It is important for Emily to seek personalised support and guidance from professionals who can assess her specific needs and provide appropriate interventions to help her navigate the academic or occupational challenges she may be facing.

2.3 Physical Signs and Symptoms

Trauma can also manifest in physical symptoms. It is important to recognise that physical symptoms can arise as a result of the physiological impact of trauma on the body. There are several common physical signs and symptoms associated with trauma.

- *Headaches and Migraines*

Chronic headaches or migraines are often reported by individuals who have experienced trauma. The persistent stress and tension associated with trauma can contribute to frequent or severe headaches.

- *Gastrointestinal Problems*

Trauma can impact the functioning of the gastrointestinal system, leading to digestive issues, such as stomach aches, nausea, diarrhoea or constipation. These symptoms may arise as a result of heightened stress and the dysregulation of the body's stress response system.

- *Fatigue and Sleep Disturbances*

The physiological and psychological impact of trauma can result in persistent fatigue and exhaustion. Sleep disturbances, such as insomnia or nightmares, can further contribute to feelings of tiredness and daytime impairment.

- *Chronic Pain and Body Aches*

Trauma can manifest as chronic pain or body aches. These physical symptoms may have no identifiable medical cause but are directly linked to the impact of trauma on the body. The heightened stress response and muscle tension associated with trauma can contribute to ongoing pain and discomfort.

- *Weakened Immune System*

Prolonged exposure to trauma can weaken the immune system, making individuals more susceptible to illnesses, and they may experience slower recovery from injuries or difficulty fighting off infections.

- *Sexual Dysfunction*

Trauma can impact an individual's sexual functioning. They may experience changes in libido, have difficulties with arousal or achieving orgasm, or feel disconnected from their bodies and sexuality.

- *Cardiovascular Problems*

The physiological impact of trauma can contribute to cardiovascular issues. Individuals who have experienced trauma may be at a higher risk of developing hypertension, heart disease or other cardiovascular conditions.

By recognising these signs and symptoms, we can better identify someone who may be struggling with the effects of trauma. It is important to approach these observations with sensitivity and empathy, understanding that each individual's experience of trauma is unique. Creating a safe and supportive environment where individuals feel comfortable discussing their experiences can foster healing and provide an opportunity for to seek the necessary help and support.

In the next chapter, we will explore the impact of trauma on different populations and discuss how trauma can intersect with various identities and experiences.

Chapter Three

Coping Strategies for
Immediate Relief

In the aftermath of a traumatic experience, individuals often find themselves grappling with overwhelming emotions, distressing memories and a profound sense of vulnerability. Coping with the trauma in this instance requires a nuanced approach that addresses both the emotional and physiological aspects of distress.

This chapter explores coping strategies designed to provide immediate relief and support individuals in navigating the early stages of their healing journey.

3.1 Grounding Techniques

Grounding techniques are designed to help individuals reconnect with the present moment, and anchor themselves when emotions and memories from the traumatic event threaten to overwhelm them. These techniques draw attention to the sensory experiences of the here and now, and serve as an effective way to interrupt distressing thoughts.

Mindfulness Meditation

Encourage individuals to engage in mindfulness meditation, where they can focus on their breath and bodily sensations. This can be done by finding a quiet space, sitting comfortably and directing attention to their breath as they inhale and exhale. When intrusive thoughts arise, gently guide attention back to the breath.

Sensory Grounding

- **5-4-3-2-1 Technique**

Guide individuals through the 5-4-3-2-1 technique as follows:

- Name five things they can see.
- Identify four things they can touch.
- Acknowledge three things they can hear.
- Recognise two things they can smell.
- Notice one thing they can taste or, if nothing is available, think about one favourite taste.

By engaging the senses, individuals ground themselves in the present moment, reducing the impact of traumatic memories.

- **Ice Cube Technique**

This technique asks the individual to hold an ice cube in their hand and describe the sensations. The cold temperature, texture and discomfort can serve as a powerful sensory experience, redirecting focus from emotional distress to the immediate physical sensations.

Visualisation

- **Safe Place Visualisation**

Guide individuals through a safe place visualisation, encouraging them to mentally create a calming and secure place and immerse themselves within it. This could be a beach or a forest, or any location where they feel safe and at ease. Encourage them to vividly imagine the sights, sounds and sensations of this safe place to foster a sense of comfort and stability.

- **Rooting Exercise**

Introduce the rooting exercise, where individuals imagine themselves as a tree with roots extending into the earth. Guide them to visualise these roots grounding them, and providing stability and strength. This visualisation promotes a sense of connection to the Earth and stability amidst emotional turbulence.

Movement-Based Grounding

- **Grounding Yoga Poses**

Introduce simple grounding yoga poses, such as the Mountain Pose or Tree Pose. These poses focus on balance, stability and connection to the earth. Guiding individuals through these movements can help bring their attention to the body and foster a sense of composure.

- **Walking Meditation**

Encourage individuals to engage in meditation as they walk, guiding them to pay attention to each step, the sensation of their feet touching the ground and the rhythmic nature of their movements. Mindful walking can promote a grounded and calm sense.

Affirmations and Mantras

- **Grounding Affirmations**

Provide individuals with grounding affirmations to repeat to themselves as they feel the need. Affirmations may include:

- "I am safe in this moment."
- "I can handle what comes my way."
- "My strength is greater than my challenges."

Repeating these affirmations can help shift mindset and provide a reassuring mental anchor.

- **Mantra Meditation**

Introduce mantra meditation, where individuals repeat a calming word or phrase. This repetition serves as a focal point, redirecting attention from distressing thoughts to the soothing rhythm of the mantra.

External Tools

- **Grounding Objects**

Suggest carrying a small grounding object, such as a 'smooth stone', a piece of fabric or a 'worry stone'. When feeling overwhelmed, individuals can hold or touch the object, focusing on its texture and weight as a tangible anchor.

- **Aromatherapy**

Explore the use of calming scents through aromatherapy. Essential oils like lavender, chamomile or cedarwood, can be applied to the skin or inhaled, providing a soothing olfactory experience that contributes to calm and stability.

Grounding techniques offer individuals immediate relief by redirecting their focus to the present moment. Visualisation, sensory engagement, movement-based practices, affirmations and external tools constitute a diverse array of grounding strategies. Tailoring these techniques to individual preferences ensures that each person can find the method that resonates most effectively with them, fostering stability and control during challenging times.

3.2 Breathing Exercises

Trauma often triggers a heightened stress response, leading to shallow breathing and increased anxiety. Breathing exercises focus on regulating the breath to promote relaxation and reduce the physiological symptoms of distress.

Diaphragmatic Breathing

Teach diaphragmatic breathing as a simple yet powerful technique. Individuals can be guided through the process via five simple steps:

1. Sit or lie down comfortably.
2. Place one hand on the chest and the other on the abdomen.
3. Inhale deeply through the nose, allowing the diaphragm to expand.
4. Exhale slowly through pursed lips, feeling the abdomen contract.
5. Repeat for several breath cycles.

Diaphragmatic breathing activates the body's relaxation response, counteracting the physiological effects of stress.

Box Breathing

Introduce the concept of box breathing, a technique commonly used for immediate stress relief. There are four simple steps:

1. Inhale for a count of four seconds.
2. Hold the breath for four seconds.
3. Exhale for four seconds.
4. Pause for four seconds before beginning the next breath cycle.

This rhythmic pattern of fours helps regulate the autonomic nervous system and promote calm.

Breathing exercises are powerful tools for managing stress, anxiety and immediate distress. These exercises focus on regulating the breath, tapping into the body's natural relaxation response and promoting a sense of calm.

Moving forward, we will explore the implementation of additional breathing exercises.

Guided Imagery Breathing

- **Beach Visualisation**

Guide individuals through a beach visualisation breathing exercise by asking them to:

1. Close their eyes and take a few deep breaths.
2. Imagine themselves on a peaceful beach.
3. Sync their breath with the rhythmic sound of ocean waves.
4. Inhale deeply as the waves roll in; exhale as they recede.

5. Continue this visualisation, focusing on the calming imagery.

This exercise combines controlled breathing with the calming effects of guided imagery.

Candle Breathing

Imagine each breath as if it were causing a candle flame to gently flicker.

Inhale slowly and deeply, visualising the flame growing taller. Exhale slowly, watching the flame subside.

This visualisation provides a tangible focal point for the breath, and aids in concentration and relaxation.

Resonant Breathing

- **Coherent Breathing**

Introduce coherent breathing. This is the practice of breathing at a rate of five breaths per minute. Individuals are guided to:

1. Inhale for a count of five seconds.
2. Exhale for a count of five seconds.
3. Continue this rhythmic breathing for several minutes.

Coherent breathing aligns with the body's natural rhythms, fostering a balanced and calming effect on the nervous system.

Alternate Nostril Breathing (Nadi Shodhana)

- **Introduction to Nadi Shodhana**

Teach individuals the technique of alternate nostril breathing, or Nadi Shodhana, to balance the two hemispheres of the brain and promote overall calmness. Follow the eight steps:

1. Sit comfortably with a straight spine.
2. Use the right thumb to close the right nostril.
3. Inhale deeply through the left nostril.

4. Close the left nostril with the right ring finger, releasing the right nostril.
5. Exhale through the right nostril.
6. Inhale through the right nostril.
7. Close the right nostril, releasing the left.
8. Exhale through the left nostril.

Repeat this cycle for several minutes, focusing on the flow of breath.

Breath Awareness Meditation

- **Mindful Breath Observation**

Guide individuals through the following breath awareness meditation:

1. Sit comfortably with eyes closed.
2. Direct attention to the natural flow of breath.
3. Observe the sensation of each inhalation and exhalation.
4. If the mind wanders, gently bring it back to the breath.

This mindfulness practice cultivates awareness of the present moment and promotes relaxation.

Breathing exercises offer a variety of techniques that individuals can choose based on their preferences and immediate needs. Visualisation, resonant breathing, alternate nostril breathing and breath awareness meditation are versatile tools that align with different comfort levels and time constraints. Encouraging individuals to explore and incorporate these exercises into their routine fosters a proactive approach to managing stress and promoting emotional wellbeing.

3.3 Progressive Muscle Relaxation (PMR)

Progressive Muscle Relaxation (PMR) is a systematic technique that involves tensing and relaxing different muscle groups in the body. This method is an effective technique to promote physical relaxation, reduce muscle tension, and alleviate the physiological symptoms of stress and anxiety. Below, we'll delve into the details of PMR and its implementation.

Guided PMR Session

Guide individuals through a progressive muscle relaxation session as follows:

1. Start with the toes, tensing the muscles for five seconds, then releasing them.
2. Move to the calves, then the thighs, and progressively work up the body.
3. Encourage participants to notice the contrast between tension and relaxation.

Regular practise of PMR can improve overall body awareness and reduce chronic muscle tension.

Extended PMR Session

- **Guided Full-body PMR**

Lead individuals through an extended PMR session that encompasses the entire body. Encourage them to:

1. Find a quiet and comfortable space to sit or lie down.
2. Starting with the toes, tense the muscles for five seconds.
3. Release the tension, allowing the muscles to relax completely for 15–20 seconds.
4. Move to the calves, then to the thighs, progressively working up the body, and including the abdomen, chest, arms and neck.
5. Encourage participants to notice the contrast between tension and relaxation in each muscle group.

This comprehensive PMR session provides a deeper sense of relaxation and can be particularly effective before sleeping.

Self-Guided PMR

Teach individuals to conduct self-guided PMR sessions. Provide a PMR script or encourage individuals to create their own. This script is useful to help individuals guide themselves through the process, focusing on specific muscle groups and allowing for relaxation between each tension phase.

Quick PMR for Stressful Moments

- **5-Minute PMR Routine**

Offer a quick and condensed version of PMR that can be done in a time-efficient manner.

1. Tense all the muscles in the hands, forearms and biceps for five seconds.
2. Release the tension for ten seconds.
3. Move to the shoulders and neck, repeating the tension and relaxation cycle.
4. Proceed to the face, including the jaw and forehead.
5. Conclude with a final tension and relaxation cycle for the entire body.

This abbreviated PMR routine provides a brief yet effective way to manage stress during a busy day.

Incorporating Breath Awareness

- **Synchronised Breathing with PMR**

Combine PMR with synchronised breathing to enhance its calming effects. Guide individuals through the following process:

1. Tense the muscles in a specific group while inhaling deeply.
2. Hold the breath for a few seconds, maintaining the tension.
3. Exhale slowly and completely, releasing the tension in the muscles.
4. Focus on the natural flow of breath between each muscle group.

Synchronised breathing adds a mindful element to PMR, and reinforces the mind-body connection.

A versatile and accessible technique, PMR can be adapted to various preferences and time constraints. Whether through guided sessions, self-guided practice or quick routines for stressful moments, PMR empowers individuals to take an active role in managing physical tension and promoting relaxation. Regular practice of PMR provides individuals with a valuable skillset for reducing stress and enhancing overall wellbeing.

3.4 Creative Expression

Creative expression is a therapeutic and empowering way for individuals to process and communicate their emotions, especially in the aftermath of trauma. Engaging in creative activities provides an outlet for self-discovery, emotional release and a tangible means of expressing complex feelings. Creative expression takes on various forms, a few of which are described below.

Art Therapy

Encourage individuals to express themselves through art. This could include drawing, painting or sculpting. The focus should be on the process rather than the end product, and allow for a release of emotions without the need for verbal articulation.

Journalling

Keeping a journal is a positive way to process thoughts and emotions. Prompts may include:

- Describe the emotions you are feeling right now
- Write a letter to yourself, offering compassion and understanding
- Capture any recurring thoughts or dreams related to the trauma.

Stream-of-Consciousness Writing

Encourage individuals to engage in stream-of-consciousness writing as a form of journaling, following these four steps:

1. Set aside a dedicated time for writing.
2. Start with a prompt or without any specific topic.
3. Write without pausing, allowing thoughts and emotions to flow freely.
4. Explore any themes or insights that emerge during the process.

Stream-of-consciousness writing can unveil deep-seated emotions and provide a cathartic release.

Gratitude Journalling

Introduce the practice of gratitude journalling. Each day, individuals jot down things they are grateful for, no matter how small. This positive focus can shift perspective and promote a sense of appreciation during challenging times.

Visual Art

- **Collage-Making**

Suggest collage-making as a visual arts activity. Provide magazines, scissors and glue, and encourage individuals to create collages that represent their emotions and aspirations, or their journey of healing. Collages can serve as visual metaphors for their experiences.

- **Vision-Boarding**

Guide individuals to create of vision boards where they collect images, words and symbols that reflect their goals, hopes and desires. Vision boards act as powerful visual reminders of what individuals want to manifest in their lives, and foster a sense of purpose and motivation.

Movement-Based Creative Expression

- **Dance and Movement**

Encourage individuals to express themselves through dance and movement. This could be free-form dance, guided dance therapy or even simple movements that feel authentic to their emotions. Movement-based expression can provide a non-verbal outlet for releasing pent-up energy and emotions.

- **Theatre and Role-Playing**

Suggest theatrical exercises or role-playing. This form of creative expression allows individuals to step into different roles and explore perspectives, providing an avenue for self-discovery and emotional exploration.

Music and Sound

- **Playlist Creation**

Encourage individuals to curate playlists that reflect their emotional landscape. Each song can represent a different facet of their experience, ultimately serving as the soundtrack to their journey. Listening to these playlists can evoke emotions and provide a sense of connection.

- **Songwriting or Poetry**

For those inclined towards writing, suggest they craft songs or poetry. Creative expression through lyrics or verse allows individuals to articulate their emotions in a structured and artistic manner. This can be a powerful means of self-expression.

Creative expression, whether through writing, visual arts, movement or music, offers individuals diverse and personalised ways to navigate their emotional landscapes. Journalling in various forms, engaging in visual arts, exploring movement-based expression and using music and sound all contribute to a holistic approach to healing. Encouraging individuals to experiment with different forms of creative expression empowers them to find the methods that resonate most deeply with their unique experiences and emotions.

3.5 Seeking Social Support

Seeking social support is a fundamental aspect of coping with trauma. Connecting with others is vital as it offers understanding, empathy and companionship during challenging times. Below are details about the forms of social support and where to seek it.

Trusted Friends and Family

Encourage individuals to reach out to friends or family members they trust. These individuals can offer a listening ear, emotional support and companionship during challenging times.

Support Groups

Suggest participation in support groups, either in-person or online, where individuals can connect with others who have experienced similar trauma. These groups provide a safe space for sharing, learning and mutual understanding.

Online Support Communities

Highlight the availability of online support communities and forums where individuals can connect with others who have experienced similar trauma. These virtual spaces offer anonymity and accessibility, allowing individuals to share their stories, ask questions and receive support from a diverse and understanding community.

Specialised Support Groups

Identify specialised support groups that cater to specific types of trauma or demographic groups. These could include groups focused on grief, domestic violence, combat veterans or other shared experiences. Specialised groups provide a more targeted and nuanced support system.

Professional Support

- **Therapeutic Support**

Emphasise the importance of seeking professional therapeutic support. Therapists, counsellors and psychologists are trained to provide a safe and confidential space for individuals to explore and process their trauma. Therapeutic interventions such as cognitive-behavioural therapy (CBT), eye movement desensitization and reprocessing (EMDR) and dialectical behaviour therapy (DBT) can be particularly effective in trauma recovery.

- **Group Therapy**

Introduce the concept of group therapy as a form of professional support. In a group setting, individuals can share their experiences, learn from others and gain insights into their healing journeys. Group therapy provides a supportive environment where individuals feel understood and less isolated.

Building and Nurturing Personal Relationships

- **Open Communication with Loved Ones**

Encourage open communication with friends and family members. Building a support network starts with expressing one's needs, fears and boundaries. Loved ones can offer emotional support, practical assistance and connection.

- **Establishing Boundaries**

Highlight the importance of establishing boundaries when seeking social support. Communicating what is helpful and what might be triggering or unhelpful is crucial. Healthy boundaries ensure individuals receive the support they need while maintaining control over their healing process.

Self-Help Groups

- **Book Clubs and Educational Groups**

Suggest joining a book club or educational group that focuses on topics related to trauma, healing and resilience. Engaging in discussions and learning together can foster a sense of community and provide valuable insights.

- **Physical Activity Groups**

Promote the benefits of joining physical activity groups or classes. Whether it is yoga, hiking or team sports, these activities contribute to physical wellbeing and provide opportunities for social connection and support.

Seeking social support is a dynamic and multifaceted process that involves connecting with others in various ways. Whether through online communities, specialised support groups, professional therapy, personal relationships or self-help groups, individuals have a range of options to build a robust support network. Encouraging individuals to explore and utilise these different avenues empowers them to create a comprehensive and personalised support system for their journey to healing.

Coping with the immediate aftermath of trauma requires a holistic approach that addresses both the emotional and the physiological aspects of distress. Grounding techniques, breathing exercises, progressive muscle relaxation, creative expression and seeking social support form a toolkit for individuals to navigate the early stages of their healing journey. These strategies empower individuals to regain control, manage distressing symptoms, and lay the foundation for deeper healing in the subsequent phases of recovery.

I Welcome Positive
Change I am open to
the positive changes
that life brings, and I
trust that these
changes will lead to
growth.

Chapter Four

Seeking Professional Help

Chapter 4 focuses on the pivotal role of professional help in healing from trauma. Seeking assistance from mental health professionals is a proactive and essential step towards understanding, processing and overcoming the impact of traumatic experiences. This chapter navigates the nuances of the therapeutic relationship, the diverse modalities of professional support and the transformative potential of counselling in the trajectory of healing.

4.1 Understanding the Importance of Professional Help

Acknowledging the Complexity of Trauma

Trauma is inherently complex due to its varied sources, manifestations and impacts on individuals. Recognising this complexity is crucial for those experiencing trauma as well as the professionals who assist them. Several key aspects underline the complexity of trauma and highlight the importance of seeking professional help.

- *Multi-dimensional Nature*

Trauma is not a singular, straightforward experience. It encompasses physical, psychological, emotional and sometimes social dimensions. For example, childhood abuse affects not only the psychological health of the individual but can also lead to physical health issues, impact social interactions and influence cognitive function.

- *Diverse Origins*

Trauma can arise from a multitude of events including natural disasters, loss of loved ones, physical or sexual abuse and witnessing violence. Each type of trauma can affect individuals in unique ways, and understanding these variances is crucial for effective treatment.

- *Variability in Response*

Individuals respond to traumatic events differently. While some might develop symptoms of PTSD, others may experience depression or anxiety, or they may experience none of these. Some might show resilience and not manifest any long-term distress. This variability necessitates a personalised approach in therapy.

- *Impact on Identity and Worldview*

Trauma can alter one's self-perception and worldview. Victims may feel a sense of betrayal, lose trust in others or develop a persistent sense of danger. Addressing these existential changes requires a deep, nuanced understanding of human psychology.

- *Secondary Traumatisation*

Sometimes, the environment around a trauma survivor can contribute to or exacerbate their condition. For instance, lack of support from family or community, stigmatisation or secondary victimisation can make recovery more challenging.

- *Potential for Re-traumatisation*

Certain interventions, if not handled sensitively, can inadvertently re-traumatise the individual. Professionals are trained to recognise these risks and navigate therapeutic interventions carefully.

Why Professional Help is Essential

Given the complexities outlined above, professional help is both beneficial and necessary for effective trauma recovery. Professionals can aid the healing process in several ways.

- *Expert Assessment*

Trained professionals can conduct thorough assessments to understand the depth and breadth of the trauma. They use validated tools and methodologies to diagnose related conditions accurately, which is crucial for effective treatment planning.

- *Tailored Treatment Plans*

Based on the assessment, professionals can create personalised treatment plans that address the specific needs, symptoms and circumstances of the individual. This might include therapies like Cognitive Behavioral Therapy (CBT), Eye Movement Desensitisation and Reprocessing (EMDR) or other appropriate interventions.

- *Safe Therapeutic Environment*

Professionals provide a safe, controlled and confidential environment where individuals can explore painful memories and emotions without judgement. This safety is crucial for effective therapy and healing.

- *Skill Building*

Beyond addressing symptoms, therapy can help individuals develop coping and resilience skills. Professionals guide clients in developing strategies to manage stress, regulate emotions and improve interpersonal relationships, which are vital for long-term recovery.

- *Support System*

Therapists often also help in building or reinforcing a support system, guiding families, friends and others to support the trauma survivor effectively.

- *Monitoring Progress*

Recovery from trauma can be a long process with ups and downs. Professionals monitor progress and can adjust treatment plans as needed, ensuring that the approach remains effective throughout the healing journey.

The path to recovery from trauma is often as complex as the experience of trauma itself. Professional help is not just a pathway to managing symptoms but a vital support in rebuilding a survivor's sense of self and control over their life. Recognising the need for professional help, and then seeking it, are crucial steps in the journey towards healing.

Breaking the silence surrounding trauma is essential. Many individuals hesitate to seek professional help due to stigma or fear of judgement. Sharing one's story in a confidential and supportive therapeutic environment is empowering.

4.2 The Therapeutic Relationship

The therapeutic relationship, often referred to as the therapeutic alliance, is a critical component of effective trauma narrative work. This relationship is the collaborative and dynamic bond between therapist and client, characterised by trust, mutual respect and agreement on therapy goals and tasks. In trauma therapy, the quality of this relationship can significantly influence the outcome of treatment. Here's a deeper exploration of its key aspects and its importance.

- Building Trust and Safety

Trust is the cornerstone of the therapeutic relationship, especially in trauma narrative work where clients must feel safe enough to explore deeply painful and personal experiences. A therapist must demonstrate consistency, empathy, confidentiality and non-judgemental understanding. Creating a safe space where clients can express their vulnerabilities without fear of retribution or misunderstanding is essential for facilitating open communication and effective treatment.

- Collaboration and Empowerment

The therapeutic relationship is inherently collaborative. Therapists and clients work together to set goals, choose therapeutic techniques and evaluate progress. This collaborative approach helps empower clients, giving them a sense of control and ownership over their healing process. It contrasts sharply with more directive or authoritarian therapeutic models, which may be less effective or even harmful in trauma work.

- Therapist's Attuneness and Responsiveness

A key element of the therapeutic relationship is the therapist's ability to be attuned to the client's emotional state and needs. This requires sensitivity to verbal cues, body language and emotional expressions, allowing the therapist to respond appropriately and adjust the pace of therapy as needed. This attunement helps clients feel understood and supported, which is crucial for building trust and facilitating deeper exploration of traumatic memories.

- Maintaining Boundaries

Effective therapeutic relationships require clear and appropriate boundaries to ensure a professional and ethical interaction. Boundaries protect both the client and the therapist and help maintain a professional relationship that is conducive to healing. This includes setting clear limits on the roles and interactions both within and outside therapy sessions.

- Handling Transference and Countertransference

Transference occurs when clients project feelings and attitudes from past relationships onto the therapist. Conversely, countertransference involves the therapist's emotional reactions to the client. These phenomena can disrupt therapy if not managed properly. Skilled therapists recognise and address transference and countertransference to avoid impairing the therapeutic relationship and to use these occurrences as therapeutic tools to delve deeper into the client's psychological landscape.

- Cultural Competence

The therapeutic relationship must be culturally competent. Therapists need to understand and respect the client's cultural background and how it influences their worldview, expressions of distress and expectations of therapy.

This understanding can enhance the therapeutic alliance by showing respect for the client's identity and integrating culturally appropriate practices.

- Continuous Evaluation

Finally, the therapeutic relationship is not static, and requires continuous evaluation and adjustment. Regular feedback sessions where clients can express their feelings about the therapy process and the relationship can help address any issues that might impact the effectiveness of therapy. This ongoing evaluation ensures the therapeutic relationship remains strong and supportive throughout the treatment process.

In trauma narrative work, the therapeutic relationship is more than just a backdrop; it is an active and potent element of the healing process. Its strength can determine the depth and success of the therapeutic engagement, making it a focal point of training and reflection for therapists specialising in trauma.

4.3 Modalities of Professional Support

Cognitive-behavioral Therapy (CBT) is a widely used and evidence-based psychotherapeutic treatment that focuses on exploring relationships between a person's thoughts, feelings, and behaviours. It is based on the cognitive model, which posits that thoughts, feelings and behaviours are interconnected and that individuals can alleviate symptoms by changing dysfunctional thoughts and behaviours.

Core Principles of CBT

- Interconnectedness of Thoughts, Feelings, and Behaviours

CBT operates on the fundamental belief that our thoughts influence our feelings, and our feelings influence our behaviours. By identifying and changing maladaptive thoughts, CBT aims to affect positive changes in emotions and behaviours.

- Focus on the Present

Unlike some forms of psychotherapy that delve into past experiences, CBT generally focuses on current problems and practical solutions to improve the individual's present state of mind.

- Structured Nature

CBT is typically more structured than other forms of therapy. Therapists often use specific agendas and techniques in each session, and treatment usually involves a limited number of sessions tailored to the client's specific goals.

- Problem-Solving Approach

CBT helps clients learn to identify and solve problems efficiently, which can reduce the symptoms of mental health conditions. The therapy focuses on teaching rational self-counselling skills.

- Goal-Oriented

CBT is goal-oriented and requires active involvement from the client. Together with the therapist, clients set specific goals at the beginning of the treatment, and these are continuously monitored and revised as needed.

Techniques Used in CBT

- Cognitive Restructuring or Reframing

This involves identifying and challenging negative thoughts or distortions and replacing them with more positive, realistic thoughts. Restructuring and reframing can change the perception of stressful situations, leading to better emotional and behavioural outcomes.

- Behavioural Activation

This technique is used primarily to combat depression. It involves encouraging clients to engage in activities they find rewarding or enjoyable, with the goal of improving their mood and interrupting patterns of depressive behaviour.

- Exposure Therapy

Often used for anxiety disorders, exposure therapy involves gradual, controlled exposure to anxiety-provoking stimuli to reduce fear or avoidance behaviours over time.

- Skill Training

This can include teaching social skills, stress management techniques and assertiveness training to help clients improve their interactions and resilience.

- Homework Assignments

CBT typically involves homework outside of therapy sessions. These assignments or practice tasks help clients apply the skills they learn in therapy to real-life situations.

Efficacy and Applications

CBT has been extensively researched and is considered highly effective for treating a variety of conditions, including depression, anxiety disorders, PTSD, eating disorders and substance abuse. It is adaptable to group, individual or family therapy formats and can be effectively delivered in in-person and teletherapy sessions.

Adaptations

CBT has been adapted to meet the needs of diverse populations and specific conditions. For example, Trauma-Focused CBT (TF-CBT) is designed specifically for individuals who have experienced trauma and addresses the unique elements of trauma symptoms and recovery.

CBT's structured, goal-oriented approach, grounded in the practical modification of thought and behaviour patterns, makes it a robust tool in the therapeutic arsenal. Its adaptability and the strong empirical support behind it continue to make it a popular choice for therapists and clients alike.

Eye Movement Desensitisation and Reprocessing (EMDR) is a distinctive psychotherapeutic approach originally designed to alleviate the distress associated with traumatic memories. Developed by Dr Francine Shapiro in 1987, EMDR has since evolved and is now used for treating various psychological issues. It is particularly noted for its effectiveness in treating PTSD.

Core Principles of EMDR

EMDR therapy is based on the premise that psychological distress is often due to disturbing life experiences that have not been adequately processed by the brain. Shapiro posited that similar to what occurs during Rapid Eye Movement (REM) sleep, bilateral stimulation such as eye movements can help the brain reprocess these frozen traumatic memories, allowing healing to occur.

The EMDR Process

EMDR therapy is typically delivered over eight distinct phases:

1. History Taking and Treatment Planning

The therapist assesses the client's history and identifies specific traumatic memories as well as current situations that cause distress. A comprehensive treatment plan is developed.

2. Preparation

The therapist ensures the client has several different ways of handling emotional distress and educates the client about the EMDR process, establishing a trust-based therapeutic relationship.

3. Assessment

The therapist identifies the vivid visual image related to the memory, a negative belief about self, related emotions and body sensations, and a positive belief. The client's baseline levels of distress are also assessed.

4. Desensitisation

The therapist leads the client in sets of bilateral stimulation, most commonly, side-to-side eye movements. After each set, the client is asked to clear their mind and notice whatever thoughts, feelings, images, memories or sensations come up, and then focus on those as the next set of bilateral movements begin. This process continues until the memory becomes less disturbing.

5. Installation

The positive belief identified in the assessment phase is strengthened and 'installed', to replace the negative beliefs.

6. Body Scan

After the client has reported no distress related to the memory, the therapist asks the client to think of the original target memory and to notice any residual somatic distress. If the client still feels tension or emotional discomfort in their body, further processing is needed.

7. Closure

The session is brought to an end whether the reprocessing is complete or not. The therapist helps the client return to a state of equilibrium using various techniques.

8. Reevaluation

At the beginning of the next session, the therapist checks to ensure the results achieved have been maintained, and then proceeds to new target memories.

Efficacy and Applications

Research has demonstrated EMDR's effectiveness for a variety of mental health conditions, particularly PTSD. Numerous studies have shown that EMDR can rapidly reduce the emotional distress stemming from traumatic memories and improve symptoms. It is also explored in treating anxiety disorders, depression and other conditions related to distressing life experiences.

Advantages and Considerations

One of the notable strengths of EMDR is its ability to achieve quick results compared to other therapeutic approaches. However, it requires specialised training and should be performed by a certified professional to ensure safety, particularly since it can initially intensify emotional reactions due to its vivid revisiting of traumatic memories.

EMDR stands out in the field of psychotherapy for its unique use of bilateral stimulation to aid the brain's natural processing abilities. It provides a structured approach to managing and overcoming trauma, and is a valuable tool in the therapeutic landscape, offering hope and healing to those plagued by the burden of traumatic memories.

Dialectical Behaviour Therapy (DBT) is a comprehensive cognitive-behavioural treatment that emphasises the psychosocial aspects of therapy. Originally developed by Dr Marsha Linehan in the late 1980s to treat individuals with borderline personality disorder (BPD) and chronic suicidal ideation, DBT has since been adapted for a variety of other mental health issues, including eating disorders, substance dependency and PTSD.

Core Principles of DBT

DBT integrates cognitive-behavioural techniques with concepts from Eastern mindfulness practices. The central dialectic within DBT is the balance between acceptance and change. Clients are taught to accept themselves as they are while also recognising the need to change unhealthy behaviours. This balance is intended to help clients increase their emotional and cognitive regulation by learning about the triggers that lead to reactive states and helping to assess which coping skills to apply in the sequence of events, thoughts, feelings and behaviours.

Key Components of DBT

DBT includes four primary modes of treatment delivery:

1. Individual Therapy

In individual sessions, therapists and clients discuss issues that come up during the week, record these on diary cards, and follow a treatment hierarchy. These sessions emphasise problem-solving for issues of all types from life-threatening behaviours to quality-of-life issues, and increasing the use of behavioural skills.

2. Group Skills Training

This component is typically conducted in a classroom setting where clients learn and practise skills alongside others. Groups meet on a weekly basis, and the entire skills curriculum is usually completed within twenty-four weeks. The skills taught are categorised into four modules: mindfulness, interpersonal effectiveness, emotion regulation and distress tolerance.

3. Phone Coaching

Clients can call their therapist between sessions to receive guidance on coping with difficult situations that arise in their everyday lives. This component supports clients in applying DBT skills in real time during actual emotional crises.

4. Consultation Team

This is a support group for the therapists themselves, providing them with a place to receive support, share experiences and ensure that treatment adheres to the DBT model. This is essential for preventing burnout among therapists and fostering effective treatment provision.

Efficacy and Applications

DBT has been empirically validated for a wide range of psychological issues. Studies have shown significant improvements in problem behaviours such as self-injury, suicidal ideation and emotional dysregulation for clients who have undergone DBT. Its applications have expanded beyond borderline personality disorder to include treatment for eating disorders, substance abuse, depression and PTSD, among others.

Distinctive Techniques in DBT

- Mindfulness

Rooted in Buddhist meditative practice, mindfulness is central to DBT and involves teaching clients how to live in the moment, develop an awareness of their thoughts and feelings, and learn to manage distress without reacting impulsively.

- Emotion Regulation

Clients are taught strategies to manage and change intense emotions that are causing problems in their lives.

- Interpersonal Effectiveness

Techniques in this module focus on strategies for asking for what one needs, saying no and coping with interpersonal conflict in a manner that is assertive, maintains self-respect and strengthens relationships.

- Distress Tolerance

This focuses on increasing a person's tolerance of negative emotion, rather than trying to escape from it, and includes handling crises and accepting life as it is in the moment.

To sum up, the structured, multi-component approach of DBT offers a powerful framework for understanding and managing emotions, improving relationships and making life-enhancing changes. Its emphasis on both acceptance and change makes it a uniquely effective therapy for disorders marked by intense emotional experiences.

4.4 Trauma-Informed Approaches

Trauma-informed approaches are an essential framework in various sectors including healthcare, social services and education. These approaches are based on the recognition of the prevalence and widespread impact of trauma, understanding how trauma can affect all individuals involved with the system and adopting a systematic approach by putting this knowledge into practice to create environments of physical, psychological and emotional safety.

Core Principles of Trauma-Informed Approaches

Trauma-informed care (TIC) is grounded in and directed by a thorough understanding of the neurological, biological, psychological and social effects of trauma and violence on humans. The key principles include:

- Safety

Ensuring physical and emotional safety for clients and providers is essential. This involves creating spaces and interactions that make individuals feel secure and respected.

- Trustworthiness and Transparency

Operations and decisions are conducted with transparency to build and maintain trust among clients, family members and staff.

- Peer Support

Peer support and mutual self-help are integral to the organisational and service delivery approach and are understood as a key vehicle for building trust, establishing safety and enabling empowerment.

- Collaboration and Mutuality

There is recognition that healing happens in relationships and the meaningful sharing of power and decision-making. The organisation recognises that everyone has a role to play in a trauma-informed approach.

- Empowerment, Voice and Choice

Throughout the organisation and among the clients served, the strengths of individuals are recognised, built on and validated, and new skills are developed as necessary. The organisation aims to strengthen the experience of choice of staff, clients and family members, and recognise that every individual's experience is unique and requires a tailored approach.

- Cultural, Historical and Gender Issues

The organisation actively moves past cultural stereotypes and biases, offers gender-responsive services, leverages the healing value of traditional cultural connections and recognises and addresses historical trauma.

Implementation in Various Settings

- Healthcare

Trauma-informed approaches in healthcare involve training staff to recognise signs of trauma in patients and interact in ways that aim to avoid re-traumatisation. This might include changes in physical spaces to feel safer and more welcoming, and procedures that give patients more control over their treatment.

- Education

Schools implementing trauma-informed approaches train teachers to recognise and respond to trauma-related behaviours. Education policies are adapted to provide a supportive environment that can address behavioural issues through a trauma-informed lens rather than punitive measures.

- Social Services

Social workers and other professionals are trained to approach clients from a perspective that considers potential trauma in their backgrounds, which might influence their behaviour and needs.

Benefits of Trauma-Informed Approaches

Adopting trauma-informed approaches can lead to several benefits including:

- Improved Client Engagement and Safety

By understanding the role trauma plays in the lives of individuals, providers can engage more effectively with those they serve and create safer service environments.

- Enhanced Client Outcomes

Trauma-informed care can lead to better client outcomes across a range of areas by addressing the root causes of issues rather than just treating symptoms.

- Reduced Rates of Re-traumatisation

Reducing re-traumatisation not only aids individual healing but can also decrease overall service use and associated costs in systems like healthcare and social services.

- Supportive Work Environments

These approaches also contribute to more supportive, sustainable and effective work environments for staff.

Trauma-informed approaches are not specific interventions but a way of structuring services, interactions and policies to help survivors of trauma feel safe, empowered and understood. By fundamentally reshaping how systems recognise and respond to trauma, these approaches foster more supportive and effective environments for both service providers and recipients.

4.5 Overcoming Barriers to Seeking Help

Addressing and overcoming barriers to seeking help for trauma is a critical aspect of mental health care. Many individuals who experience trauma do not seek the support they need due to a variety of obstacles. Understanding and addressing these barriers can significantly enhance the accessibility and effectiveness of trauma-related services.

Common Barriers to Seeking Help

- Stigma and Shame

Many cultures stigmatise mental health issues, which can lead to feelings of shame or embarrassment about seeking help. Individuals may fear judgement from others or believe that seeking help is a sign of weakness.

- Lack of Awareness

Some individuals may not recognise the signs of trauma or may not know their experiences qualify as traumatic. Others may not be aware of the services available to them or how those services might help.

- Financial Constraints

Therapy and other mental health services can be expensive, and not all services are covered by insurance. This financial burden can be a significant deterrent, especially for those without insurance or with limited financial resources.

- Fear of Reliving Trauma

The process of healing from trauma often involves discussing past traumatic experiences, which can be a daunting prospect. Fear of re-traumatisation or distress at reliving painful memories can prevent individuals from engaging in therapy.

- Cultural and Linguistic Barriers

For individuals from different cultural backgrounds, particularly those for whom English is a second language, finding services that accommodate their language and respect their cultural context can be challenging. Cultural misunderstandings between clients and therapists can also hinder effective treatment.

- Logistical Issues

Practical issues such as lack of transport, inflexible work schedules or caregiving responsibilities can impede access to treatment.

- Lack of Trust

Mistrust in the healthcare system, often due to past negative experiences or systemic biases, can deter individuals from seeking help.

Strategies to Overcome Barriers

- Increasing Mental Health Awareness

Community education programs that explain what trauma is, its effects and the benefits of seeking treatment can help reduce stigma and raise awareness. Media campaigns, workshops and school programs can be effective tools.

- Making Services More Accessible

Sliding scale fees, insurance coverage and free community services can make help more financially accessible. Teletherapy and mobile health options can also reduce logistical barriers by allowing individuals to receive care from home.

- Cultural Competence in Therapy

Training therapists to be culturally competent can help bridge the cultural and linguistic gaps. Offering services in multiple languages and hiring therapists from diverse backgrounds can also make mental health care more accessible and effective.

- Building Trust

Programs designed to build or rebuild trust in healthcare providers can be crucial. This might involve community outreach, integrating respected community members into the health promotion process and ensuring transparency in treatment practices.

- Peer Support

Support groups, especially those led by peers who have experienced and overcome similar trauma, can be particularly effective in reducing stigma and fear. These groups provide a sense of community and mutual understanding that can be very encouraging for those hesitant to seek help.

- Education on Coping Mechanisms

Teaching coping mechanisms as part of the therapy process can help individuals manage the stress of reliving traumatic memories, making the prospect of therapy less daunting.

Overcoming barriers to seeking help for trauma is essential to ensure all individuals can heal and recover. By addressing these barriers through comprehensive strategies at individual, community and systemic levels, mental health services can become more inclusive, effective and supportive. This not only benefits those directly affected by trauma but also contributes to the overall health and wellbeing of the community.

Chapter Five

Processing Trauma Through Narrative

Trauma, whether experienced in a single moment or endured over an extended period, leaves an indelible mark on an individual's psyche. The process of healing from trauma is complex, often involving the integration of fragmented memories, emotional upheavals and a reconstruction of one's sense of self. One powerful avenue for this healing is through narrative therapy, where individuals articulate and reshape their experiences into coherent, empowering stories.

In this chapter, we delve into the profound role of narrative in processing trauma, exploring the therapeutic journey of turning pain into a narrative of resilience, growth and transformation.

5.1 Understanding Trauma Narratives

Defining Trauma Narratives: Unravelling the Threads of Experience

Trauma narratives are the intricate stories individuals weave to make sense of experiences that have deeply impacted their psychological and emotional wellbeing. These narratives go beyond a mere chronological account of events; they are the emotional and cognitive rendering of a person's journey through trauma. To define trauma narratives, it is essential to explore their multifaceted nature to understand the interplay between memory, language and the reconstruction of a fractured sense of self.

The Complexity of Trauma Stories

Trauma narratives are not linear or straightforward. Unlike a conventional narrative arc, trauma stories often lack a clear beginning, middle and end. They might be fragmented, disjointed or marked by gaps in memory, reflecting the disruptive nature of traumatic experiences on the narrative structure. Understanding this complexity requires therapists and individuals alike to navigate through layers of emotion, cognition and sensory impressions.

Beyond Explicit Details: The Implicit Dimensions

While explicit details of a traumatic event may find their way into a narrative, the implicit dimensions of trauma stories are equally significant. Implicit elements encompass the unspoken emotions, somatic sensations and unarticulated aspects of the experience. These implicit dimensions often carry immense emotional weight, shaping the emotional tone and impact of the narrative.

Memory as a Shifting Canvas

Memory, a central element in any narrative, takes on a unique character in the context of a trauma narrative. The very nature of traumatic events can impact memory recall, leading to fragmented or distorted recollections. Defining a trauma narrative involves recognising that memory is not a static entity but a dynamic, evolving canvas influenced by the interplay of time, emotion and subsequent experiences.

Language as a Medium of Expression

The choice of language becomes crucial in defining a trauma narrative. Individuals may grapple with finding words to articulate the inexpressible aspects of their trauma. The selection of words, metaphors and symbols becomes a nuanced process as individuals attempt to convey the depth of their emotional experience. This linguistic exploration is not just a tool for expression but an integral part of the therapeutic process.

The Nuances of Narrative Construction

Trauma narratives are constructed with a palette of emotions, perceptions and interpretations. The storyteller becomes both the narrator and the protagonist, recounting not only the events but the internal struggles, coping mechanisms and transformations. This process involves weaving together disparate threads into a coherent tapestry that reflects the individual's unique journey through trauma.

Cognitive Reorganisation: Making Sense of Chaos

One of the defining features of a trauma narrative is the cognitive reorganisation that occurs during the storytelling process. Individuals grapple with making meaning out of chaos, imposing a semblance of order on experiences that may initially seem incomprehensible. This cognitive reorganisation is not just a retrospective act but an ongoing, dynamic process as individuals continually reinterpret and reconstruct their narratives.

Emotional Resonance: Beyond the Facts

Trauma narratives carry a profound emotional resonance that extends beyond the factual details of an event. The emotions embedded in the narrative — grief, fear, anger, resilience — become a vital part of its definition. Therapists working with trauma narratives pay careful attention to the emotional texture of the story, understanding that the affective elements often hold the key to unlocking deeper layers of meaning.

Sensory Impressions: The Texture of Experience

Trauma is not just a cognitive or emotional experience, but also a sensory one. Defining a trauma narrative involves acknowledging the sensory impressions woven into the fabric of the story. The therapist listens both to what is said as well as the texture of the experience — the sights, sounds, smells and bodily sensations that contribute to the richness of the narrative.

The Interplay Between Silence and Utterance

Defining a trauma narrative requires exploration of the interplay between silence and utterance. Trauma often introduces moments of unspeakable pain, where words fail to capture the depth of the experience. Therapists guide individuals through the delicate dance of finding language for the unsaid, recognising that silence itself is a potent element in the narrative.

Unspoken Trauma: The Language of Silence

Trauma narratives frequently grapple with the challenge of articulating the inarticulable. Silence becomes a language of its own — a space where unspoken pain, shame or fear resides. Therapists create a safe container for individuals to navigate this silence, understanding that the absence of words is as meaningful as their presence.

Finding Utterance: Giving Voice to Experience

Conversely, defining a trauma narrative involves empowering the individual to find a voice for their experiences. This process is not just about speaking the facts but about giving voice to the emotional truths that may have been suppressed or denied. Therapists encourage individuals to use language as a tool for reclaiming agency and authorship over their stories.

The Healing Potential of Expression

Expression, whether in words, art or any other form, holds an immense healing potential in trauma narratives. Utterance becomes a bridge between the internal world of the individual and the external world of shared meaning. Through this process, individuals move beyond the isolation of their experiences, finding connection and understanding.

The Role of Narrative in Identity Reconstruction

Trauma narratives play a pivotal role in the reconstruction of identity. Defining oneself in the aftermath of trauma involves integrating the narrative of the past into the evolving story of the present and future. This process involves recounting events and shaping a narrative that fosters resilience, agency and a sense of self beyond victimhood.

From Victim to Survivor: Shifting Narratives of Identity

One of the transformative aspects of a trauma narrative is the potential to shift from the narrative of victimhood to one of survivorship. Therapists collaborate with individuals to reframe their experiences, emphasising strengths, coping strategies and moments of resilience. This shift in narrative identity is not a denial of the pain but a reclamation of agency and power.

Narrative Coherence: Creating a Sense of Order

Defining trauma narratives involves the pursuit of narrative coherence — the order and meaning that helps individuals make sense of their experiences. Therapists guide individuals as they identify the threads that contribute to coherence, whether through themes of growth, self-discovery or the triumph of the human spirit over adversity.

Narrative Flexibility: Embracing Multifaceted Identities

Trauma narratives are not static; they evolve and adapt as individuals grow and change. Defining the trauma narrative involves embracing narrative flexibility, and recognising that identity is multifaceted and can encompass both the scars of the past and the possibilities of the future. This narrative flexibility is a testament to the inherent resilience within humans and our capacity for growth and adaptation.

Exploring the trauma narrative allows individuals to uncover the nuanced and intricate process of storytelling in the aftermath of trauma. These narratives are not just accounts of past events; they are living, breathing expressions of the human spirit's resilience and capacity for growth. Therapists engaged in this work navigate the delicate terrain of memory, language and identity, guiding individuals toward narratives that empower, heal and foster a sense of agency in the ongoing journey towards recovery.

The Multifaceted Nature of Trauma Stories: Beyond Chronology

The telling of trauma stories is a complex and nuanced process that goes beyond merely recounting events in chronological order. To truly grasp the multifaceted nature of trauma stories, it is crucial to explore the layers of emotion, meaning and sensory experiences that individuals bring to their narrative. When we unravel the intricacies of a trauma story, we can understand how they are woven from threads of memory, emotion and the interplay between the explicit and implicit dimensions.

Layers of Emotional Complexity

Trauma stories are rich tapestries of emotion. Emotions infuse every aspect of the narrative, creating a spectrum of feelings, ranging from profound sorrow and fear to resilience and hope. Understanding these layers of emotional complexity involves recognising that each emotion contributes to the texture of the story, shaping its impact on the storyteller and the listener.

Expressive and Repressed Emotions: The Duality of Experience

In each trauma story, there is a duality of expressive and repressed emotions. Some emotions find direct expression in the narrative, vividly coloring recounts of events. However, other emotions often remain beneath the surface, hidden in the recesses of the storyteller's psyche. Therapists navigate this duality, creating a space for both overt and covert emotions to find expression.

The Evolution of Emotional Themes: From Despair to Resilience

Trauma stories evolve emotionally, much like the human experience itself. What might begin as a narrative steeped in despair can transform into one marked by resilience and triumph. Therapists guide individuals through the exploration of these emotional themes, helping them understand how their emotions have shifted and how new emotional threads have been woven into the narrative over time.

The Implicit Dimensions of Trauma Stories

While explicit details of traumatic events find their way into a narrative, it is the implicit dimensions that add depth and nuance. Implicit elements include unspoken emotions, sensory impressions and embodied experiences that often evade direct articulation. Understanding the implicit dimensions is akin to deciphering the unsaid, recognising that there is often profound meaning in what is not explicitly mentioned.

The Unspoken Senses: Engaging the Body in the Story

Trauma is a sensory experience that goes beyond words. The sensations — the tightening of the chest, the churning stomach, the racing heartbeat — are implicit in trauma stories. Therapists encourage individuals to bring these sensations into the narrative, recognising that the body holds a significant role in the storytelling process.

Symbolic Imagery: Metaphors and Representations

Trauma stories often employ symbolic imagery as individuals grapple with finding language for the ineffable. Metaphors, symbols and representations become powerful tools for expressing aspects of the experience that resist direct articulation. Therapists guide individuals to explore the symbolic dimensions of their stories, understanding that the use of metaphor can unveil layers of meaning.

Memory as a Shifting Mosaic

Memory, a cornerstone of narrative construction, takes on a dynamic and shifting character in trauma stories. The chronological unfolding of events may not align neatly with the progression of memory recall. Instead, memory is a mosaic — a collection of fragmented pieces that individuals work to piece together as they recount their experiences.

Fragmentation and Gaps: The Challenge of Memory Recall

Traumatic events can fragment memory, creating gaps and distortions in the narrative. These gaps are not just omissions; they represent the areas where the emotional impact of the trauma may be too overwhelming for direct articulation. Therapists navigate these gaps with sensitivity, recognising that memory recall is an ongoing process that may evolve throughout the therapeutic journey.

The Influence of Time: How Memory Shifts Over the Years

The passage of time influences the nature of memory in trauma stories. What might be vividly remembered in the immediate aftermath of a traumatic event can undergo shifts in emphasis and significance over the years. Therapists guide individuals to explore how time has shaped their memories, understanding that the narrative is not a fixed entity but an evolving reflection of their experiences.

Language as a Medium of Expression

The choice of language becomes a critical element in the multifaceted nature of trauma stories. Language is not merely a tool for communication, it is a medium through which individuals give shape to their experiences, emotions and the complexities of their inner worlds.

The Search for Words: Articulating the Inexpressible

Individuals often grapple with finding words for the inexpressible aspects of their trauma. Therapists foster an environment where individuals feel supported in their search for language, recognising that the process of articulation itself is a significant aspect of the therapeutic journey.

Narrative Style: The Tone and Texture of Expression

Trauma stories unfold in varied narrative styles. Some individuals may adopt a factual and detached tone, while others express their stories with intense emotion. The narrative style is not just a matter of personal preference; it reflects the storyteller's relationship with their experiences and the emotional weight they carry.

The Therapeutic Role of Exploring Multifaceted Trauma Stories

The exploration of the multifaceted nature of trauma stories is not merely an intellectual exercise; it is a therapeutic endeavour with profound implications for the healing process.

Validation and Recognition: Affirming the Complexity of Experience

In delving into the emotional, implicit and linguistic dimensions of trauma stories, therapists offer validation and recognition. Affirming the complexity of experience communicates to individuals that their stories are not reducible to a linear sequence of events; rather, they are intricate expressions of the human response to trauma.

Facilitating Integration: Weaving Threads into a Coherent Whole

The therapeutic process facilitates the integration of fragmented elements into a coherent whole. Therapists guide individuals to weave the threads of emotion, memory and language into a narrative that fosters a sense of understanding, resilience and agency.

Empowerment Through Expression: Reclaiming Agency in the Story

Exploring the multifaceted nature of trauma stories is an empowering process. It allows individuals to reclaim agency in their narratives, recognising that their stories are not dictated solely by the traumatic events but by the meaning-making process that unfolds in the therapeutic space.

In understanding the multifaceted nature of trauma stories, therapists embark on a journey that goes beyond the surface of events. They navigate the emotional terrain, explore the implicit dimensions and appreciate the intricacies of memory and language. Through this exploration, each individual finds a platform for expression, validation and integration — a space where their story, with all its complexity, contributes to the process of healing and resilience.

Trauma stories are multifaceted, reflecting the complexity of the human experience. They encompass not only the explicit details of the traumatic event but also the implicit, often unspoken, dimensions of pain. Exploring trauma narratives requires a sensitivity to both the overt and covert aspects of the story, acknowledging that the unsaid might carry as much weight as the spoken.

The Role of Memory in Trauma Narratives: Weaving Threads of the Past

Memory, a dynamic and complex construct, plays a pivotal role in the creation and articulation of trauma narratives. When individuals recount their experiences of trauma, they are not just recalling a series of events but engaging with the complex interplay of memory, emotion, and cognition. This section delves into the nuanced role of memory in trauma narratives, unravelling the threads that weave the past into the present narrative.

Understanding the Complexity of Memory

Memory is not a static archive of past events but a dynamic and reconstructive process. In the context of trauma, where the impact on the individual is profound, memory takes on unique characteristics that influence the storytelling process.

Fragmentation and Gaps in Memory Recall

Traumatic events can lead to fragmentation and gaps in memory. The sheer intensity of emotions during traumatic experiences can disrupt the encoding and consolidation of memories, resulting in fragmented recall. There may be gaps in the narrative; areas where memory seems elusive or inaccessible. These gaps are not indicative of forgetfulness but rather represent the areas where the emotional weight of the trauma may be too overwhelming for direct articulation.

Influence of Emotional Salience on Memory

Emotional salience, the degree to which an event is emotionally charged, profoundly shapes memory. Traumatic events are etched into memory with heightened emotional intensity, making them more likely to be retained and recalled vividly. The emotional impact of trauma not only affects the encoding of memories but also influences the subsequent retrieval and reconstruction of those memories.

The Role of Intrusive Memories in Trauma

Intrusive memories, characterised by involuntary and vivid recall of traumatic events, are a distinctive feature of trauma. These memories can surface unexpectedly, triggered by stimuli that may bear no apparent connection to the traumatic event. The interplay between intrusive memories and the narrative construction process is a complex one, with therapists guiding individuals in navigating the emotional challenges posed by these involuntary recollections.

The Shifting Landscape of Traumatic Memory

Memory of traumatic events is not fixed, it is subject to shifts and alterations over time. The process of memory recall is influenced by myriad factors, including the passage of time, subsequent life experiences and the individual's evolving cognitive and emotional state.

Temporal Aspects: How Time Shapes Memory

The temporal aspects of memory are crucial in understanding the shifting landscape of traumatic recall. Memories of trauma may change emphasis, significance or emotional tone as time passes. What was initially remembered with vivid detail may gradually become a part of a broader narrative, with the impact of time acting as a nuanced storyteller.

Integration of Subsequent Experiences

Subsequent life experiences become integrated into the narrative of traumatic memory. Individuals may find that their understanding of the traumatic event evolves as they encounter new challenges, engage in therapy or build relationships. Therapists assist individuals in recognising how subsequent experiences can shape the narrative, contributing to a more comprehensive understanding of the trauma.

Coping Mechanisms and Memory Modification

Coping mechanisms, ranging from avoidance to active engagement, influence the modification of traumatic memories. Some individuals may employ strategies to avoid thinking about or discussing the traumatic event, while others may actively seek to confront and integrate the memories. The role of coping mechanisms in memory modification underscores the intricate relationship between the individual's cognitive processes and emotional wellbeing.

Challenges in Memory Recall: Gaps and Inconsistencies

The process of recalling traumatic memories is fraught with challenges, leading to gaps, inconsistencies and variations in narrative detail. Understanding these challenges is essential for therapists working with trauma narratives.

Cognitive Biases in Memory Recall

Cognitive biases can impact the accuracy of memory recall. Individuals may experience cognitive distortions, such as selective attention or memory amplification, where certain aspects of the traumatic event are emphasised while others are minimised or overlooked. Therapists employ techniques to mitigate these biases and foster a more accurate recall of the traumatic event.

Repression and Retrieval Blockades

Repression, a defence mechanism where the mind actively suppresses distressing memories, can create retrieval blockades. Individuals may encounter difficulty accessing certain aspects of the traumatic event due to repression. Therapists work delicately to create a safe space for individuals to explore repressed memories, recognising that the process requires trust and a gradual unfolding of narrative details.

Variability in Narrative Detail: The Nature of Traumatic Memory

The variability in narrative detail is intrinsic to the nature of traumatic memory. Individuals may provide inconsistent accounts of the same event, and the narrative may evolve. This variability is not indicative of dishonesty or fabrication but reflects the inherent complexity of trauma and the challenges associated with recounting distressing experiences.

Memory as a Source of Empowerment: The Therapeutic Aspect

While memory poses challenges in the articulation of trauma narratives, it is also a potent source of empowerment and healing. Therapists leverage the therapeutic aspect of memory to facilitate the individual's journey toward understanding, acceptance and resilience.

Validation Through Memory Recall

Memory recall offers a form of validation for individuals who may have experienced doubt or disbelief regarding their traumatic experiences. As memories are articulated and shared, bearing witness becomes a powerful validation of the individual's reality. Therapists play a crucial role in affirming the significance of memory in the validation process.

Reconstructing the Narrative: From Fragmentation to Coherence

The therapeutic process involves reconstructing the narrative from the fragments of memory. Therapists guide individuals in weaving together the threads of memory, filling gaps and creating a coherent and meaningful account of their traumatic experiences. This process is not about imposing a linear structure but about fostering a narrative that aligns with the individual's sense of self and understanding.

The Integration of Emotional and Cognitive Processes

Memory recall in the therapeutic context integrates both emotional and cognitive processes. Therapists recognise that memory is not a purely intellectual exercise but a deeply emotional one. Encouraging individuals to explore the emotional dimensions of their memories fosters a more comprehensive understanding of the trauma and its impact on their lives.

The Ethical Dimensions of Memory Work in Trauma Therapy

Engaging with memory in trauma therapy raises ethical considerations that therapists must navigate with sensitivity and care. The very act of recalling traumatic memories can be emotionally taxing, and therapists must prioritise the wellbeing of individuals throughout the therapeutic process.

Informed Consent and Autonomy

Informed consent is a foundational ethical principle in memory work. Therapists ensure that individuals fully understand the nature of memory exploration, the potential emotional challenges and the voluntary nature of their participation. Respecting autonomy is paramount, and individuals are empowered to decide the pace and depth of their engagement with memory recall.

Addressing Potential Retraumatisation Risks

Memory work carries the risk of retraumatisation, where the act of recalling traumatic events exacerbates distress. Therapists closely monitor for signs of emotional overwhelm and employ strategies to mitigate potential risks. The goal is to create a therapeutic environment that is supportive, validating and attuned to the individual's emotional wellbeing.

Cultural Sensitivity and Diverse Perspectives on Memory

Cultural sensitivity is integral to the ethical practice of memory work. Therapists recognise that cultural norms, beliefs and practices influence an individual's perspective on memory and storytelling. Approaching memory work with cultural humility ensures the therapeutic process is inclusive and respects diverse ways of engaging with and expressing traumatic memories.

Future Directions: Memory, Technology and Therapeutic Innovation

The evolving landscape of technology introduces new dimensions to the exploration of memory in trauma therapy. From virtual reality to digital platforms, technological advancements offer innovative ways to engage with memory recall and narrative construction.

Virtual Reality and Memory Recontextualisation

Virtual Reality (VR) technology provides a unique opportunity to recontextualise traumatic memories. Therapists explore the potential of VR in creating immersive environments where individuals can revisit and reshape their memories. The dynamic nature of VR allows for a more interactive and participatory approach to memory work.

Digital Storytelling Platforms and Narrative Expression

Digital storytelling platforms offer individuals diverse ways to express their narratives. Individuals can construct narratives that extend beyond traditional verbal articulation through multimedia elements, such as images, audio and video. Therapists explore the integration of digital storytelling into the therapeutic process, recognising the potential for creative and personalised expression.

Ethical Considerations in Technology-Assisted Memory Work

As technology is integrated further into trauma therapy, ethical considerations take centre stage. Therapists navigate questions of privacy, data security and the potential impact of technology on the therapeutic relationship. Ensuring that technological interventions align with ethical principles is crucial in exploring memory in trauma therapy.

Memory as a Tapestry of Resilience

In the intricate tapestry of trauma narratives, memory is the thread that weaves the past into the present, shaping the narrative landscape of an individual's life. From the fragmented recollections of traumatic events to the dynamic shifts over time, memory is both a challenge and a source of empowerment in the therapeutic process. Therapists navigate the complexities with sensitivity, recognising that each memory, whether vivid or elusive, contributes to the rich and resilient tapestry of the human experience. In the exploration of memory within trauma narratives, individuals find not just a recounting of the past but a pathway towards understanding, healing and reclaiming agency over their own stories.

Memory, a central element in narrative construction, operates differently in the aftermath of trauma. The fragmented and sometimes disjointed nature of traumatic memories challenge the linear narrative structure. Exploring how memory functions in the trauma narrative is crucial for therapists and individuals alike, as it influences the coherency and emotional resonance of the story.

5.2 The Therapeutic Power of Storytelling: Illuminating Paths to Healing

Storytelling is a fundamental human impulse, a way we make sense of the world, share experiences and connect with others. In trauma, storytelling takes on a unique and potent therapeutic role. This section delves into the multifaceted dimensions of the therapeutic power of storytelling, examining how narratives unfold, shape and ultimately contribute to the healing journey.

The Inherent Human Need for Storytelling

Storytelling is deeply ingrained in the human experience. From ancient oral traditions to modern digital platforms, humans have been telling stories as a means of communication, to preserve culture and, importantly, as a way to navigate the complexities of life. This intrinsic human need for storytelling forms the foundation for its therapeutic potential.

The Evolutionary Significance of Storytelling

The evolutionary significance of storytelling lies in its role in the transmission of knowledge, culture and survival strategies across generations. Through stories, communities passed down essential information about navigating their environment, dealing with adversity and finding meaning in their existence. In the therapeutic context, this evolutionary aspect is harnessed to explore and navigate the landscape of trauma.

Storytelling as Meaning-Making

At its core, storytelling is an act of making meaning. Humans instinctively seek to make sense of their experiences, especially those that are distressing or traumatic. Through narrative construction, individuals impose order on the chaos of their internal world, creating a framework within which they can understand, process and integrate the impact of trauma on their lives.

Connection Through Shared Narratives

In sharing stories of trauma, individuals not only communicate their personal experiences but also tap into the universal aspects of human suffering. These shared narratives create connection and understanding and reduce the isolation often associated with traumatic experiences.

The Unique Role of Storytelling in Trauma Recovery

In the context of trauma recovery, storytelling serves as a dynamic and multifaceted tool. Therapists harness the power of narratives to facilitate exploration, expression and, ultimately, the transformation of the traumatic experience into a coherent and meaningful story.

Narrative Exposure as a Therapeutic Process

Narrative exposure is a therapeutic process through which individuals are guided to construct a coherent narrative of their traumatic experiences. This process involves recalling and recounting the traumatic event within the therapeutic space, providing a structured framework for the exploration of emotions, memories and the meaning ascribed to the trauma.

Externalisation of Trauma Through Storytelling

Storytelling externalises the trauma, allowing individuals to distance themselves from overwhelming emotions and experiences. By framing the traumatic event as a narrative, individuals gain a sense of authorship and agency over their story, reducing the emotional immediacy that can cause the overwhelm.

Reconstruction of Identity Through Narrative

Trauma often fractures one's sense of identity. Storytelling becomes a vehicle for the reconstruction of identity, allowing individuals to weave the narrative threads of their past, present and future into a cohesive and evolving sense of self. The act of narrating one's story becomes an intentional and transformative process.

The Neurobiology of Storytelling and Healing

The therapeutic power of storytelling is not confined to the realm of psychology; it extends into the neurobiological processes of the brain. Storytelling engages various brain regions, releasing neurochemicals that play a crucial role in emotional regulation and resilience.

Oxytocin and the Social-Emotional Bond

Oxytocin, often referred to as the 'bonding hormone', is released during social interactions, including storytelling. The act of sharing one's narrative in a supportive and empathetic environment triggers the release of oxytocin. In turn, this fosters connection, trust and emotional bonding between the storyteller and the listener. In the therapeutic relationship, this neurobiological response contributes to the establishment of a secure and trusting space.

Dopamine and the Reward System

The brain's reward system, mediated by the release of dopamine, is activated during engaging and meaningful experiences, including storytelling. When individuals find resonance in their narratives — whether through self-discovery, validation or the expression of resilience — the reward system is activated. This neurobiological response reinforces the therapeutic process, making storytelling an inherently rewarding and motivating aspect of trauma recovery.

Cortisol Regulation and Stress Reduction

Storytelling contributes to the regulation of cortisol, the stress hormone. Engaging in narrative therapy allows individuals to express and process their emotions, reducing the physiological stress response associated with trauma. Through articulating their stories, individuals move from a state of heightened arousal to a calmer and more regulated emotional state.

Narrative Therapy Techniques in Trauma Recovery

Narrative therapy encompasses a variety of techniques that therapists employ to facilitate the therapeutic power of storytelling. These techniques are designed to support individuals to explore their narratives, reconstruct meaning and foster resilience.

Externalisation and Objectification

Externalisation involves separating the individual from the problem or trauma, allowing them to view it as an external entity. Objectification goes a step further by giving the trauma a physical form or representation. These techniques assist in creating a tangible and manageable distance between the individual and their traumatic experiences, enabling a more objective exploration.

Reauthoring and Rewriting the Narrative

Reauthoring involves revisiting and rewriting aspects of the narrative to emphasise strengths, resilience and growth. Therapists collaborate with individuals to challenge negative or disempowering aspects of their stories, fostering a more positive and adaptive narrative. This process of rewriting contributes to the reconstruction of identity and the cultivation of a sense of agency.

Witnessing and Validating Narratives

The therapeutic relationship provides a space for witnessing and validating narratives. Therapists actively listen, empathise and acknowledge the emotional and cognitive dimensions of the individual's story. This process of witnessing and validation is transformative, as it affirms the individual's reality, fosters a sense of connection, and contributes to the restoration of agency.

Creative Expression and Storytelling

Creative expression serves as a powerful complement to verbal storytelling in trauma recovery. The use of art, writing, music and other forms of creative expression provides individuals with an alternative means of articulating their experiences, emotions and the complexities of their trauma narratives.

Art Therapy as Visual Storytelling

Art therapy allows individuals to narrate their experiences visually. Through painting, drawing or sculpting, individuals can externalise and explore their trauma in a non-verbal manner. The visual narrative becomes a parallel storytelling process, offering insights and expressions that may not be easily conveyed through words alone.

Writing and Journalling as Narrative Exploration

Writing and journalling provide individuals with a private space for narrative exploration. Putting pen to paper becomes a form of self-reflection and expression. Therapists often encourage individuals to maintain journals to track the evolution of their narratives, observe patterns and engage in a continuous process of meaning-making.

Music and Movement as Embodied Narratives

Music and movement serve as embodied narratives, allowing individuals to express and explore their emotions through non-verbal channels. Therapists incorporate music therapy and movement-based interventions to enhance the expressive possibilities of storytelling. These modalities engage the body in the narrative process, recognising the integral connection between the physical and emotional dimensions of trauma.

Cultural Considerations in Storytelling and Healing

Storytelling is deeply influenced by cultural contexts, norms and traditions. In the therapeutic space, cultural considerations play a crucial role in how individuals engage with and express their narratives. Therapists adopt a culturally sensitive approach to storytelling, recognising the diverse ways in which trauma is perceived, articulated and healed across different cultural frameworks.

Cultural Narratives and Healing Practices

Cultural narratives, myths and healing practices shape an individual's perspectives on trauma and recovery. Therapists collaborate with individuals to integrate cultural narratives into their personal stories, recognising the significance of cultural identity in the healing process. This inclusive approach ensures that the therapeutic journey respects and aligns with diverse cultural perspectives.

Language and Symbolism in Cultural Storytelling

Language and symbolism hold cultural significance in storytelling. Therapists acknowledge the diversity of linguistic expression and symbolic meaning embedded in cultural narratives. Language becomes a bridge between personal and cultural storytelling, allowing individuals to articulate their experiences within the rich tapestry of their cultural contexts.

Challenges and Considerations in Trauma Storytelling

While storytelling is a powerful tool in trauma recovery, it is not without its challenges. Therapists navigate ethical considerations, potential retraumatisation risks and the complexities of working with narratives that may be fragmented or elusive.

Ethical Considerations in Trauma Storytelling

Ethical considerations in trauma storytelling centre around issues of consent, confidentiality and the individual's wellbeing. Therapists prioritise informed consent, ensuring that individuals understand the process of narrative exploration, potential emotional challenges and the voluntary nature of their participation. Confidentiality safeguards the privacy of the individual's story and therapists uphold ethical standards in the responsible use of narrative material.

Addressing Retraumatisation Risks

Storytelling carries the inherent risk of retraumatisation, where the act of recalling a traumatic event can exacerbate distress. Therapists closely monitor for signs of emotional overwhelm and employ strategies to mitigate potential retraumatisation risks. This involves creating a safe and supportive therapeutic environment, respecting the individual's pacing and incorporating trauma-informed approaches.

Balancing Fragmented Narratives

Traumatic experiences can result in fragmented narratives, where memories are disjointed, incomplete or inconsistent. Therapists approach fragmented narratives with sensitivity, recognising that gaps may exist due to the nature of trauma. The therapeutic process involves navigating these gaps collaboratively, allowing individuals to share what feels safe and gradually expanding the narrative as trust is built.

Future Directions: Technology, Narratives and Healing

The intersection of technology and storytelling opens new avenues for trauma recovery. From virtual reality interventions to digital platforms for narrative expression, technological advancements offer innovative tools for therapists and individuals engaging in the therapeutic power of storytelling.

Virtual Reality (VR) and Immersive Narratives

Virtual reality (VR) technology provides opportunities for immersive storytelling experiences. Therapists explore the potential of VR to create virtual environments where individuals can engage with and recontextualise their narratives. The immersive nature of VR enhances the therapeutic impact of storytelling, offering a unique platform for exploration and healing.

Digital Platforms for Narrative Sharing

Digital platforms provide individuals with diverse mediums for narrative sharing. Blogs, podcasts and social media platforms offer spaces for individuals to share their stories with a broader audience, fostering a sense of community and reducing the stigma associated with trauma. Therapists navigate the ethical considerations of online storytelling, ensuring the protection of privacy and wellbeing.

Artificial Intelligence (AI) and Personalised Narratives

Artificial intelligence (AI) holds potential in the development of personalised narrative interventions. AI algorithms can analyse patterns in an individual's narrative, offering insights into emotional states, cognitive processes and areas of focus for therapeutic exploration. The integration of AI into narrative therapy opens avenues for more tailored and responsive interventions.

Illuminating Paths to Healing Through Storytelling

In the intricate tapestry of trauma recovery, storytelling emerges as a guiding light, illuminating paths to healing, resilience and self-discovery. From the ancient traditions of oral storytelling to the modern, technologically augmented narratives of today, the act of sharing and shaping stories remains a fundamental aspect of the human experience.

In the therapeutic context, storytelling is not merely a recounting of the past; it is a dynamic and transformative process. Through narrative exploration, individuals navigate the landscape of trauma, externalize their experiences, and reconstruct meaning. The therapeutic power of storytelling extends beyond the verbal domain, embracing creative expressions and cultural narratives that contribute to the richness of the healing journey.

Therapists, as facilitators of these narratives, navigate the complexities with sensitivity, ethical consideration and a profound understanding of the neurobiological and cultural dimensions of storytelling. In each shared story, a journey unfolds — one that leads from the shadows of trauma into the light of resilience, empowerment and a renewed sense of self. Through the therapeutic power of storytelling, individuals not only reclaim their narratives but also embark on a profound voyage of healing, where the stories they tell are a testament to the strength of the human spirit.

5.3 Cultural and Social Dimensions of Trauma Narratives

Trauma is a complex and deeply personal experience that is, in many ways, shaped by cultural and social contexts. The telling of trauma narratives – the stories individuals construct to make sense of their traumatic experiences – is inherently influenced by cultural norms, societal attitudes and collective histories. This exploration delves into the intricate interplay between culture, society and trauma narratives, recognising that understanding these dimensions is essential for a comprehensive grasp of the impact of trauma.

The Cultural Construction of Trauma Narratives

Cultural Variations in Expressing Trauma

Different cultures have unique ways of expressing and conceptualising trauma. The cultural lens through which individuals view their experiences influences not only the content of their trauma narratives but also the emotional tone and the perceived implications of the trauma. For example, in some cultures, stoicism and silence may be culturally valued, impacting how trauma is communicated and shared.

Language and Linguistic Nuances

The language used to articulate trauma is deeply embedded in cultural nuances. Certain cultures may have specific terms or idioms that capture the essence of trauma in ways that transcend mere translation. Understanding these linguistic nuances is crucial for professionals working in diverse cultural contexts to ensure the richness of the narrative is preserved.

Cultural Symbols and Metaphors

Cultural symbols and metaphors play a significant role in trauma narratives. A traumatic experience might be likened to a journey, a battle or a descent into darkness, and these metaphors carry cultural meanings that shape the narrative. The symbolism attached to certain images or events can be deeply ingrained in cultural narratives and collective memory.

Societal Influences on the Construction of Trauma Narratives

Stigmatisation and Silence

Societal attitudes towards trauma can either facilitate or impede the construction of trauma narratives. In cultures where there is a stigma attached to discussing trauma or mental health issues, individuals may be more inclined to silence their narratives. Understanding the societal dynamics that contribute to this silence is crucial for creating spaces to encourage openness and healing.

Power Dynamics and Marginalised Voices

The power dynamics within a society can significantly impact whose trauma narratives are acknowledged and validated. Marginalised groups may find their stories dismissed or overlooked. Recognising and addressing these power imbalances is essential for creating an inclusive and equitable environment where all voices can be heard.

Societal Memory and Collective Trauma

Societal memory, shaped by historical events and collective traumas, influences how individuals situate their personal narratives within a broader context. Historical trauma, such as war or systemic injustice, cast long shadows on the narratives of individuals and communities. Acknowledging and addressing collective trauma is integral to understanding the layers of meaning within trauma narratives.

Intersections of Culture, Identity and Trauma

Cultural Identity and Intersectionality

Individuals hold intersecting identities shaped by factors such as culture, race, gender and sexual orientation. These intersecting identities profoundly influence the construction and interpretation of the trauma narrative. For example, one person's experience of trauma as a member of a minority group may be fundamentally different from that of a person in the majority.

Cultural Competence in Trauma-Informed Care

Cultural competence in trauma-informed care requires an understanding of how cultural factors intersect with trauma experiences. Professionals must be attuned to the nuances of cultural identity, ensuring that interventions are sensitive to the cultural context and don't inadvertently perpetuate harm or reinforce cultural stereotypes.

Immigration, Acculturation and Trauma

For individuals who have migrated, the experience of trauma is often entwined with the challenges of acculturation. Trauma narratives for immigrants may involve a complex interplay between the trauma experienced in their country of origin and the stressors associated with adapting to a new culture. Understanding this intersection is crucial for providing effective support.

Rituals, Healing and Cultural Practices

Rituals as Narrative Structures

Cultures often have rituals and ceremonies that serve as structured narratives for processing and healing from trauma. These rituals can be deeply symbolic, providing a framework for individuals to make meaning of their experiences. Integrating these cultural practices into therapeutic interventions can enhance the healing process.

Cultural Approaches to Resilience

Cultural narratives of resilience and coping strategies play a vital role in trauma recovery. Understanding how different cultures conceptualise and cultivate resilience can provide valuable insights for developing culturally sensitive interventions. Some cultures may draw on spiritual practices, community support or traditional healing methods as integral components of resilience.

The Role of Community in Healing

In many cultures, healing from trauma is a communal endeavour. The community's support, whether through family structure, religious institutions or other social networks, is integral to the healing process. Recognising the communal dimensions of trauma narratives is essential for developing interventions that acknowledge and leverage these social supports.

Challenges and Considerations in Cross-Cultural Trauma Work

Ethical Considerations in Cross-Cultural Settings

Working with trauma narratives across diverse cultures requires a deep commitment to ethical practice. Professionals must be aware of cultural sensitivities, power dynamics and potential biases in their approach. This involves ongoing self-reflection, cultural humility and a willingness to learn from and with the individuals they serve.

Translation and Interpretation Challenges

Language nuances can be challenging to translate accurately, and the cultural context can impact the interpretation of translated narratives. Utilising skilled interpreters and translators who understand both the language and cultural subtleties is crucial for maintaining the integrity of trauma narratives.

Addressing Cultural Stigma and Barriers to Help-Seeking

Cultural stigma surrounding mental health and trauma can be a significant barrier to seeking help. Trauma-informed approaches need to include strategies for reducing stigma and fostering a cultural understanding of mental health that encourages help-seeking.

Future Directions: Towards Culturally Responsive Trauma Care

Integrating Cultural Competence in Training Programs

Training programs for mental health professionals need to incorporate cultural competence as a core component. This includes education on diverse cultural perspectives on trauma, strategies for culturally sensitive communication and an awareness of the social determinants that impact trauma experiences.

Research on Culturally Tailored Interventions

Further research is needed to explore the effectiveness of culturally tailored interventions for trauma. This involves investigating how interventions can be adapted to align with cultural values, beliefs and practices while maintaining fidelity to evidence-based practices.

Advocacy for Inclusive Policies and Services

Advocacy efforts are essential for promoting inclusive policies and services that consider the cultural and social dimensions of trauma. This includes advocating for diversity in mental health services, addressing systemic barriers and promoting cultural competence at institutional levels.

A Culturally Informed Approach to Trauma Narratives

Understanding the cultural and social dimensions of trauma narratives is not just an academic exercise but a crucial aspect of providing effective and compassionate care. Culturally informed approaches recognise the diversity of human experience and honour the unique ways an individual navigates their trauma. By embracing cultural competence, professionals contribute to creating a more inclusive and equitable landscape for healing from trauma; one that respects and integrates the richness of diverse narratives.

5.4 Challenges in Narrative Processing

Narrative processing – the act of making sense of and giving meaning to one's experiences through storytelling – is a complex and often challenging aspect of trauma recovery. While narratives can be powerful tools for healing, they are not without their difficulties. This exploration delves into the challenges inherent in narrative processing, understanding that navigating these hurdles is integral to the therapeutic journey.

Fragmentation and Incomplete Stories

The Puzzle of Memory

One significant challenge in narrative processing arises from the fragmented nature of memory, especially in the aftermath of trauma. Traumatic events can disrupt the normal encoding and consolidation of memories, leading to fragmented recollections. This fragmentation can result in individuals struggling to construct cohesive and linear narratives.

Gaps and Ambiguities

Trauma often leaves gaps and ambiguities in one's narrative. Some details may be vividly remembered, while others remain obscured or distorted. These gaps can create challenges in constructing a comprehensive and coherent narrative. Therapists must navigate these spaces delicately, acknowledging the limitations of memory.

Emotional Intensity and Avoidance

Overwhelm and Emotional Flood

Narrative processing can evoke intense emotions associated with the traumatic event. Revisiting and recounting these experiences may lead to emotional overwhelm, making it challenging for individuals to articulate their stories coherently. Therapists must create a safe space for expression, while helping individuals manage the emotional intensity that narrative processing can unleash.

Avoidance and Silence

Conversely, individuals may engage in avoidance behaviours, resisting or suppressing the narrative process. This avoidance can manifest as reluctance to share certain details, a preference for vague language or a complete withdrawal from narrative processing. Unpacking the reasons behind avoidance is a delicate task for therapists.

Shifting Perspectives and Meaning-Making

Changing Interpretations Over Time

Trauma narratives are not static; they evolve over time as individuals gain new perspectives and insights. A challenge arises when the meaning attributed to the traumatic event shifts, sometimes leading to confusion or a need to reevaluate the narrative. Therapists must be attuned to these shifts and support individuals in their evolving meaning-making process.

Balancing Multiple Narratives

In cases involving interpersonal trauma, individuals may grapple with the challenge of balancing their narratives with those of others involved. Navigating the complexities of multiple perspectives, especially in situations of conflicting accounts, requires sensitivity and skill on the part of the therapist.

Shame, Guilt and Self-Blame

The Weight of Shame and Guilt

Trauma narratives often carry the heavy burdens of shame and guilt. Individuals may grapple with feelings of responsibility for the traumatic event or harbour a sense of shame about their reactions or perceived vulnerabilities. Addressing these elements within the narrative requires a delicate and non-judgemental therapeutic approach.

Unravelling Self-Blame Narratives

Self-blame narratives can become deeply ingrained in the trauma story. Individuals may construct narratives where they attribute blame to themselves, even in situations where external circumstances or other individuals were responsible. Unravelling these self-blame narratives necessitates careful exploration and reframing.

Linguistic and Cultural Challenges

Language Limitations

The expression of trauma is inherently tied to language, and linguistic challenges can impede the narrative process. This is especially relevant in cross-cultural contexts where nuances may be lost in translation and certain concepts may lack direct equivalents. Therapists need to be aware of these language limitations and employ creative communication strategies.

Cultural Taboos and Sensitivities

Cultural considerations can pose challenges, particularly when certain topics are considered taboo or highly sensitive within a specific cultural context. Therapists must navigate these cultural nuances with respect and cultural competence, ensuring that the narrative process aligns with the individual's cultural framework.

External Pressures and Judgement

Fear of Stigmatisation

External factors, such as societal stigma or judgement, can significantly impact the narrative process. Individuals may fear societal reactions to their trauma narratives, leading to self-censorship or a reluctance to disclose certain details. Therapists play a crucial role in mitigating these fears and creating a confidential and non-judgemental therapeutic space.

Legal Implications

In cases where trauma is connected to legal matters, individuals may be cautious about the potential legal implications of their narratives. Fear of legal consequences can hinder open and honest disclosure. Therapists need to be aware of the legal framework and work collaboratively with individuals to navigate these concerns.

Reconstructing a Sense of Agency

Reclaiming Narrative Agency

Trauma can profoundly impact an individual's sense of control. The process of narrative processing involves not only recounting the traumatic event but also reclaiming a sense of agency in shaping one's narrative. Therapists assist individuals in reconstructing a narrative that emphasises resilience, coping and a forward-looking perspective.

Empowering Through Narratives

Empowering individuals through their narratives involves highlighting moments of strength, resilience and survival. Therapists actively collaborate with individuals to identify and amplify these elements within the narrative, contributing to a sense of empowerment and mastery over one's life story.

Navigating the Complexities of Narrative Processing

While narrative processing is a potent tool for healing, it is not a straightforward or linear journey. Therapists must navigate the intricate web of the memories, emotions, cultural influences and societal dynamics that shape trauma narratives. Recognising and addressing the challenges inherent in narrative processing is essential for creating a therapeutic space that fosters resilience, growth and a renewed sense of self. It is through these challenges that individuals, with the support of skilled therapists, can embark on a transformative journey of healing and meaning-making.

5.5 Case Studies: Narratives of Resilience

Below, we explore several case studies that highlight the resilience shown by individuals as they process their trauma narratives.

Case Study 1: Overcoming Childhood Abuse

Anna, a 30-year-old woman, entered therapy to deal with the emotional scars left by a childhood marred by physical and emotional abuse. Through narrative therapy, Anna learned to articulate her experiences, which she had never verbally expressed. Initially, her stories were fragmented and filled with self-blame. Over time, and through guided therapeutic techniques,

Anna began to reframe her narrative, recognising her younger self's strength and resilience. She gradually shifted from seeing herself as a victim to acknowledging herself as a survivor who had navigated tremendous hardships. This shift significantly improved her self-esteem and helped her establish healthier interpersonal relationships.

Case Study 2: Recovering from a Violent Assault

James, a 40-year-old male, was struggling with PTSD following a violent assault. He found it particularly challenging to talk about the incident without experiencing severe anxiety and flashbacks. Through the use of narrative exposure therapy, James and his therapist worked together to create a chronological account of his life, placing the traumatic event within the larger context of his life story. This process helped James to contextualise the trauma, reducing its overwhelming impact. By the end of the therapy, James was able to narrate his experience with significantly reduced distress and began to view his response to the assault as a testament to his resilience and ability to endure.

Case Study 3: Healing from the Loss of a Loved One

Maria, a 55-year-old woman, sought therapy after the sudden death of her spouse. The loss had left her debilitated with grief and isolated from her social circles. Through narrative therapy, Maria slowly began to articulate her deep sense of loss and the love she had for her spouse. By processing these emotions, she began to see her continued life as a tribute to the love she and her spouse shared. This perspective allowed her to engage with her grief without being consumed by it, and she eventually found new ways to connect with others who had experienced similar losses, fostering a sense of community and shared resilience.

Case Study 4: Confronting and Overcoming Addiction

David, a 28-year-old, had battled drug addiction for a decade. His addiction was initially triggered by an attempt to cope with unresolved childhood neglect. Narrative therapy was pivotal in his recovery process. By recounting his life story, David identified patterns and triggers of his substance abuse. Recognising the link between his emotional neglect and his addiction helped him to develop more effective coping mechanisms. As David reshaped his narrative from one of neglect to one of self-awareness and recovery, he rebuilt his life, reestablished estranged relationships and pursued a career in counselling to help others with similar struggles.

Case Study 5: Rebuilding Trust After Marital Betrayal

Ethan, a 45-year-old man, entered therapy feeling disillusioned and betrayed after discovering his spouse's long-term affair. The betrayal had shattered his trust and left him questioning his self-worth and the validity of his past experiences. Ethan struggled with intense feelings of anger, confusion, and sadness. Through narrative therapy, Ethan began articulating his feelings and experiences surrounding the betrayal. Early sessions focused on allowing him to express his pain without judgement, helping him externalise and organise the tumultuous emotions he was dealing with. As therapy progressed, Ethan worked with his therapist to reframe his narrative, focusing on his resilience and capacity for forgiveness, rather than seeing himself solely as a victim of his spouse's actions.

One significant breakthrough occurred when Ethan was encouraged to explore the broader context of his life, including his strengths and achievements outside of his marriage. This helped him realise that while the betrayal was a part of his story, it did not define his entire life or his value as a person. By acknowledging his resilience in facing previous life challenges, Ethan began to see himself as a strong individual capable of overcoming adversity. Moreover, narrative processing allowed Ethan to reconstruct his view of the relationship and his future. He worked on redefining his personal goals and values, separate from his identity as a partner. This redefinition was crucial for his healing process, allowing him to make informed decisions about how to move forward, either by working towards reconciliation with his spouse or by building a new life for himself.

Ethan's therapy journey highlighted the importance of narrative in recovering from personal betrayal. By re-authoring his life story to emphasise his resilience and capacity for growth, Ethan regained confidence in his ability to trust and build meaningful relationships in the future. This case study underscores how narrative therapy can be a powerful tool in recovering from the deep emotional wounds caused by marital betrayal, facilitating a transformative journey from hurt to healing and empowerment.

These case studies demonstrate the power of narrative processing in building resilience among trauma survivors. By reinterpreting their traumatic experiences within a new, empowering narrative framework, individuals can transform their understanding of themselves and their past, leading to healing and personal growth. This therapeutic approach not only helps individuals cope with past trauma but also enhances their capacity to navigate future challenges with increased resilience and confidence.

5.6 Ethical Considerations in Trauma Narrative Work

Informed Consent and Boundaries

Engaging in trauma narrative work requires careful attention to ethical considerations. Informed consent is crucial, with therapists ensuring individuals fully understand the process and potential emotional challenges. Establishing and maintaining boundaries is equally vital in creating a safe therapeutic space.

Cultural Sensitivity and Diversity

Cultural sensitivity and diversity are pivotal aspects of ethical practice in trauma narrative work. Trauma is experienced, expressed and processed through the lens of an individual's cultural background, which profoundly impacts the therapeutic approach and effectiveness. Understanding and respecting cultural differences is not just an ethical obligation but a necessary component of effective therapy.

Let's explore why cultural sensitivity and diversity are crucial in more detail.

Understanding Cultural Expressions of Trauma

Different cultures have varied ways of expressing and dealing with trauma. For example, some cultures might emphasise stoicism and discourage overt emotional expressions, while others might encourage sharing and emotional expression as a way of healing. A therapist must be attuned to these differences to interpret a client's reactions accurately and provide support that respects the client's cultural expressions of distress.

Respecting Cultural Healing Practices

Many cultures have traditional healing practices and rituals that play a significant role in coping with trauma. Integrating these practices into the therapeutic process can enhance comfort and trust, and potentially increase the efficacy of treatment. Therapists should show respect for these practices and explore ways to respectfully incorporate them into treatment plans, if appropriate and desired by the client.

Avoiding Cultural Assumptions

Therapists must avoid making assumptions based on a client's cultural background. This involves recognising and setting aside one's own biases and preconceptions. Making assumptions can lead to misunderstandings and can compromise the effectiveness of therapy. It is important for therapists to engage in continuous cultural competence training and to approach each client's situation with openness and humility.

Language and Communication Styles

Effective communication is key in trauma narrative work, and language barriers or differences in communication style can pose significant challenges. Therapists should be aware of the nuances in communication styles across different cultures and consider the use of interpreters or culturally familiar co-therapists when necessary. Additionally, non-verbal communication can vary significantly between cultures, and understanding these differences is crucial for building rapport and trust.

Ethical Consideration of Power Dynamics

Cultural sensitivity also involves an awareness of the power dynamics that can exist when a therapist and client come from different cultural or socioeconomic backgrounds. Therapists must strive to equalise the inherent power imbalances in the therapeutic relationship by empowering clients and validating their cultural identities and experiences.

Collaboration with Community Resources

Engaging with community leaders and resources can enhance cultural sensitivity in therapy. These resources can provide valuable insights into the client's cultural background and current community dynamics. Collaboration can also help make the therapy more accessible and acceptable within specific cultural contexts.

Continued Education and Self-Reflection

Therapists must commit to ongoing education about cultural diversity and regular self-reflection on their own cultural identities and biases. This ongoing learning helps therapists stay informed about the best practices in culturally competent care and ensures they continue to improve their ability to serve diverse populations effectively.

Cultural sensitivity and diversity in trauma narrative work are not just ethical imperatives but foundational aspects that significantly influence the therapeutic outcome. By embracing cultural competence, therapists can provide a more empathetic, respectful and effective therapeutic environment, leading to better outcomes for clients dealing with trauma.

Addressing Retraumatisation Risks

Re-traumatisation is a critical concern in trauma narrative work, where the act of recounting traumatic experiences might inadvertently lead to a resurgence of trauma symptoms. This can include emotional distress, physiological responses like panic attacks, or a re-emergence of post-traumatic stress disorder (PTSD) symptoms. Addressing the risks of re-traumatisation is not only a crucial aspect of effective therapy but also an ethical imperative to do no harm.

Let's take a deeper look at how to mitigate these risks in therapeutic settings.

Gradual Exposure

One of the fundamental techniques to minimise the risk of re-traumatisation is to ensure that the recounting of traumatic events is approached gradually. Therapists often use techniques like titration, which involves slowly and carefully exposing a client to the traumatic memory, ensuring it does not overwhelm their current coping mechanisms. This method allows the client to progressively build resilience and emotional tolerance.

Creating a Safe Space

Before delving into trauma narratives, it's crucial to establish a strong therapeutic alliance and a safe, supportive environment for the client. This includes clear communication about the process and goals of therapy, establishing trust and ensuring the client feels in control of their narrative and the pace at which it unfolds.

Stabilisation Techniques

Prior to engaging in detailed trauma narratives, therapists often work with clients to develop stabilisation and grounding techniques. These skills are crucial for clients to manage potential distress effectively. Techniques might include mindfulness, deep breathing or sensory awareness exercises that help keep the client anchored in the present moment if memories become overwhelming.

Client Empowerment

Ensuring that clients feel a sense of empowerment is vital in preventing re-traumatisation. This involves letting them make informed decisions about their therapeutic journey, including when and how to share their trauma narrative. Empowerment also involves reinforcing their strengths and resilience, highlighting their ability to survive and to cope with their past experiences.

Monitoring and Adjusting

Continuous monitoring of the client's emotional and psychological state during sessions is essential. Therapists must be attuned to any signs of distress and be prepared to adjust the approach accordingly. This could mean taking a break from the trauma narrative, revisiting stabilisation techniques or possibly postponing the narrative work until the client feels more resilient.

Post-Session Support

Providing support after sessions that involve intense trauma work is crucial. This can include follow-up calls, making sure the client has a supportive environment to return to, or equipping them with strategies to manage any delayed reactions to discussing traumatic events.

Therapist Self-Care

Addressing re-traumatisation is not only about client care but also about therapist self-care. Therapists can be vicariously traumatised through exposure to trauma narratives, which can impact their ability to provide safe and effective therapy. Regular supervision, peer support and personal therapy can help therapists manage their emotional responses and maintain their professional effectiveness.

Feedback Mechanisms

Incorporating regular feedback mechanisms into the therapy process can help identify early signs of re-traumatisation. This involves asking clients directly about their experience of the sessions, any distress they felt and their perceptions of safety within the therapeutic relationship.

Addressing the risk of re-traumatisation requires a careful, thoughtful and client-centred approach. By implementing these strategies, therapists can help ensure that trauma narrative work serves as a path to healing rather than a source of further trauma.

5.7 Future Directions in Trauma Narrative Research

As the field of trauma therapy continues to evolve, the exploration of trauma narrative work is poised at a crucial juncture, ripe for innovative advancements and deeper inquiries. The next phase of research in this domain aims to expand our understanding of the mechanisms through which narrative processing affects healing and to refine techniques to maximise therapeutic outcomes for diverse populations.

This chapter on will delve into emerging trends, potential technological integrations and cross-disciplinary approaches that enhance the efficacy and reach of trauma narrative therapies. By addressing existing gaps and exploring new methodologies, this research will not only deepen our theoretical knowledge but also improve practical applications, ultimately fostering more nuanced and effective trauma care.

Advancements in Neuroscience and Trauma Narratives

The intersection of neuroscience and trauma narratives represents a burgeoning field of study that offers insights into how trauma is encoded and processed, and how it can be effectively treated in the human brain. Recent advancements in neuroscience have begun to elucidate the neural mechanisms underlying the therapeutic effects of narrative work, providing a biological basis for practices that have been used clinically for years.

Let's take a deeper look into these advancements and their implications for trauma therapy.

Brain Plasticity and Narrative Therapy

One of the most critical contributions of neuroscience to trauma therapy is the concept of neuroplasticity — the brain's ability to reorganise itself by forming new neural connections throughout life. This adaptability is at the core of narrative therapy's effectiveness. Recounting and restructuring trauma narratives can lead to changes in how traumatic memories are stored and processed in the brain. Research suggests that reshaping a trauma narrative can help move the memory from the amygdala (associated with emotional reactions) to the prefrontal cortex (involved in rational thought), thereby reducing the immediate, visceral impact of traumatic memories.

Mapping Emotional Processing

Functional MRI (fMRI) studies have shown that engaging with trauma narratives activates specific brain areas, including the hippocampus, amygdala and prefrontal cortex. Understanding these activation patterns helps clinicians see how trauma impacts brain function and guides them in developing targeted interventions that can help rewire these neural pathways, promoting recovery from trauma.

Stress Response and Narrative Expression

Neuroscience research has highlighted the role of the hypothalamic-pituitary-adrenal (HPA) axis in the stress response, which is often dysregulated in individuals with PTSD. Narrative therapy can help regulate this response, as articulating trauma can diminish the physiological stress reactions over time, thereby alleviating symptoms of hyperarousal and anxiety.

Neurobiological Correlates of Resilience

Studies are increasingly focusing on understanding the neurobiological correlates of resilience — the capacity to recover quickly from difficulties, which is a critical aspect of effective trauma therapy. Insights into the neural foundations of resilience can inform narrative approaches by identifying specific narrative elements that strengthen resilience pathways in the brain.

Integration of Biofeedback

Leveraging technological advancements, some narrative therapies now incorporate biofeedback mechanisms to provide real-time data on physiological responses (like heart rate and skin conductance) during therapy sessions. This integration allows for a more nuanced understanding of how recounting certain aspects of trauma affects the body, enabling therapists to tailor interventions more precisely and effectively.

Personalised Therapy through Neuroimaging

Future research aims to use neuroimaging techniques to predict individual responses to different types of narrative therapy. This approach could lead to more personalised therapy, where treatment modalities are tailored not just to the psychological profile of the patient but also to their neurobiological characteristics.

Longitudinal Studies

Long-term neuroscience research following individuals through the course of narrative therapy can provide valuable insights into how narrative changes impact brain function over time. These studies are crucial for understanding the enduring effects of narrative work on brain structure and function.

The fusion of neuroscience and narrative therapy for trauma opens up exciting possibilities for both understanding and treating trauma more effectively. As this field advances, it holds the promise of offering more refined, personalised, and scientifically grounded therapeutic options to those grappling with the aftermath of traumatic experiences. This ongoing convergence of neuroscience and psychological practice not only enhances therapeutic techniques but also deepens our understanding of the human experience of trauma and resilience.

Technology and Narrative Processing

The integration of technology into narrative processing for trauma therapy represents a significant advancement in the field, enhancing the accessibility, efficacy, and personalization of treatments. Technological tools ranging from virtual reality (VR) to artificial intelligence (AI) are reshaping how narratives are explored and processed in therapeutic settings.

Let's take a look at the key technological innovations and their impact on trauma narrative work.

VR Therapy

VR technology has been increasingly utilised to create immersive therapeutic environments where patients can safely confront and reprocess traumatic memories. In VR settings, therapists can control the environment completely, allowing for gradual exposure to trauma triggers in a controlled and safe manner. This can help patients re-encounter the traumatic event and engage with their narrative in a way that reduces fear and anxiety, under the careful guidance of a therapist.

AI in Narrative Analysis

AI technologies, including natural language processing (NLP), are being used to analyse trauma narratives in more depth. These tools can help identify patterns, themes and emotional tones in the narratives that might be difficult for human therapists to discern consistently. AI can provide insights into the progression of therapy, suggest areas that need more focus, and even help customise therapeutic interventions based on the linguistic cues found in patient narratives.

Digital Storytelling Tools

Various apps and software platforms allow individuals to create digital stories involving text, images and sounds. These tools give patients new ways to express their narratives, particularly for those who may find verbal expression challenging. Digital storytelling can be a powerful medium for articulating complex trauma narratives and can be particularly engaging for younger clients or those from tech-savvy generations.

Teletherapy and Narrative Sharing

The rise of teletherapy platforms has made trauma therapy more accessible to those who might not be able to attend in-person sessions due to geographical, physical or psychological barriers. These platforms often include features like secure video conferencing and digital journals, allowing for ongoing narrative work that is both flexible and confidential. Additionally, these tools can facilitate group therapy sessions, providing a space for sharing narratives with others who have similar experiences, thereby reducing feelings of isolation.

Biofeedback and Neurofeedback

These technologies use sensors to provide real-time feedback about physiological states, such as heart rate, brain activity and muscle tension. This feedback can help patients become more aware of their bodily responses when recounting trauma narratives and learn to control these responses through relaxation techniques, enhancing the therapeutic process.

Mobile Apps for Continuous Support

Mobile applications can provide ongoing support and guidance for individuals engaged in narrative processing. These apps may include features like reminders for narrative writing, mood tracking, coping skill tutorials, and prompts for reflection. They serve as an adjunct to traditional therapy, offering continuous engagement and support, which is crucial for managing trauma symptoms effectively.

The incorporation of technology into narrative processing for trauma therapy is opening new frontiers for treatment modalities, making therapy more personalised, engaging and accessible. As these technologies continue to evolve, they promise to enhance our understanding of trauma and expand the tools available for its effective treatment. This marriage of technology and narrative therapy not only democratises access to mental health services but also deepens the therapeutic impact by embracing innovations that cater to the unique needs of trauma survivors.

In the intricate tapestry of trauma and healing, narratives serve as both the threads of pain and the stitches of resilience. This chapter has journeyed through the terrain of trauma narratives, emphasising their complexity, therapeutic potential and cultural dimensions. From the principles of narrative therapy to the challenges, ethical considerations and future directions in research, the exploration of trauma through narrative is a dynamic and evolving field. As we conclude this chapter, we recognise the transformative power of stories—their ability to heal, empower and ultimately rewrite the narrative of survival and growth after trauma.

My journey is
unique, and so is
my pace. I respect
my process and
trust in my timing

Chapter Six

✤

Building Resilience and Post-Traumatic Growth

Chapter 6 explores the practical strategies and mindset shifts necessary for building resilience in the face of life's challenges. Resilience is not just a trait but a skill that can be cultivated through intentional practices and perspectives.

This chapter aims to empower individuals with tools to navigate adversity, bounce back from setbacks and foster a mindset that promotes long-term wellbeing.

6.1 Understanding Resilience

The Dynamic Nature of Resilience: An Ever-Evolving Skill

Resilience is not a static quality but a dynamic and evolving skill that individuals can actively cultivate throughout their lives. This understanding of resilience as a dynamic process involves recognising its fluidity, adaptability and continuous capacity for growth.

Let's take a closer look at the key aspects of the dynamic nature of resilience.

Adaptability in the Face of Adversity

Resilience involves the ability to adapt in the face of adversity. Life is inherently unpredictable and challenges come in various forms. A resilient mindset is not about avoiding difficulties but about developing the flexibility to navigate them successfully. It's the art of adjusting the sails when the winds of life change direction.

Continuous Learning and Growth

Resilience is intertwined with a commitment to continuous learning and personal growth. Individuals who embrace resilience see challenges not as insurmountable obstacles but as opportunities for learning and development. Every setback becomes a stepping stone for personal evolution, contributing to an ongoing journey of self-discovery.

Shifting Perspectives on Setbacks

The dynamic nature of resilience is evident in how individuals perceive and respond to setbacks. Resilient individuals develop a growth mindset in which setbacks are reframed as opportunities for improvement, rather than as indicators of personal failure. This shift in perspective is crucial for maintaining a positive outlook in the face of adversity.

Building a Resilient Mindset Over Time

Developing resilience is a gradual and cumulative process. It's not a quality that one possesses or lacks; rather, it's a mindset that is honed over time through experiences, reflections and intentional efforts. The more individuals consciously engage with challenges and setbacks, the more resilient their mindset becomes.

Resilience Across the Lifespan

Resilience is applicable at every stage of life. It's not a trait reserved for certain age groups or life situations. Children, adolescents, adults and older individuals can all benefit from cultivating resilience. The skills and attitudes that contribute to resilience may evolve, but the essence of bouncing back and adapting remains constant.

Cultivating Resilience Through Various Strategies

The dynamic nature of resilience is evident in the myriad strategies individuals can use to cultivate it. From mindfulness practices to positive habits, social connections and problem-solving skills, resilience can be nurtured through a diverse range of approaches. This adaptability ensures that individuals can find strategies that resonate with their unique preferences and circumstances.

Resilience as a Process, Not a Destination

Understanding the dynamic nature of resilience involves recognising that it's a process rather than a destination. There's no fixed endpoint where one achieves 'ultimate resilience'. Instead, it's an ongoing journey marked by progress, setbacks and continual refinement of one's ability to face life's challenges.

Community and Collective Resilience

Resilience extends beyond individual capacities to community and collective levels. Societies and communities that foster a culture of support, inclusion and adaptability are inherently more resilient. Recognising the interconnectedness of individual and collective resilience highlights the societal impact of cultivating this dynamic skill.

Reflection and Iteration

Reflection plays a vital role in the dynamic nature of resilience. Individuals who actively reflect on their experiences, setbacks and coping mechanisms gain insights that contribute to the refinement of their resilience. This process of reflection and iteration ensures individuals continually adapt and refine their approaches to challenges.

The dynamic nature of resilience underscores its capacity for growth, adaptability and continuous development. Recognising resilience as a dynamic skill empowers individuals to actively engage with life's challenges, viewing them as opportunities for learning and personal evolution. By understanding that resilience is a process, not a fixed trait, individuals can approach setbacks with a mindset that fosters adaptability, strength and an enduring commitment to self-improvement.

The Role of Mindset: Nurturing Resilience Through Perspectives

The role of mindset in resilience is foundational, shaping how individuals perceive, interpret and respond to life's challenges. It's not just about the events themselves but about the perspectives individuals adopt in the face of adversity. Understanding and cultivating the right mindset is crucial for building and strengthening resilience.

Shifting to a Growth Mindset

The concept of a growth mindset was introduced and popularised by psychologist Carol Dweck in her book Mindset: The New Psychology of Success. In this book, first published in 2006, Dweck explores the distinction between what she terms "fixed" and "growth" mindsets. She argues that adopting a growth mindset—the belief that abilities and intelligence can be developed through effort, learning, and persistence—can lead to increased motivation and achievement. This concept has since been widely influential in various fields including education, psychology, and business.

Individuals with a growth mindset view challenges as opportunities to learn and grow, rather than as insurmountable obstacles.

Cultivating a growth mindset involves three key factors:

- Embracing challenge – resilient individuals embrace challenges as chances to stretch their abilities.
- Seeing effort as a path to mastery – effort is seen not as fruitless but as a pathway to mastery and improvement.
- Learning from criticism – constructive feedback is viewed as valuable input for growth, rather than a personal attack.

Embracing Change

Resilient individuals approach change with a positive and adaptable mindset. Instead of resisting or fearing change, they view it as an inherent part of life. This perspective enables them to navigate uncertainties with a sense of flexibility and openness.

Mindset shifts for embracing change include:

- Viewing change as inevitable – recognising that change is a constant in life, resilient individuals accept it rather than resist it.
- Focusing on adaptability – emphasising the importance of adapting to new circumstances fosters a proactive approach to change.
- Finding opportunities in change – resilient individuals look for opportunities for growth and learning within the context of change.

Learning from Setbacks

Resilient individuals approach setbacks with a mindset geared towards learning and improvement. Instead of viewing failures as indicators of personal inadequacy, they see them as stepping stones on the path to success.

Mindset shifts for learning from setbacks include:

- Seeing setbacks as temporary – resilient individuals view setbacks as temporary challenges, rather than permanent failures.
- Analysing and adapting – the focus is on analysing what went wrong, adapting strategies and using setbacks as learning opportunities.
- Understanding the value of persistence – a resilient mindset understands that persistence is key; setbacks are not the end, but part of a longer journey.

Building Resilience Over Time

Resilience is not an overnight achievement but a continuous process. The mindset towards building resilience involves a commitment to ongoing personal development, acknowledging that the journey towards greater resilience is a gradual one.

Mindset shifts for building resilience over time include:

- Setting realistic expectations – resilient individuals set realistic expectations for their progress, and understand that building resilience is a journey with ups and downs.
- Celebrating progress – small victories are celebrated as indicators of progress, reinforcing the idea that resilience is built incrementally.
- Embracing the journey – the focus is not solely on reaching a destination but on embracing the ongoing journey of self-discovery and growth.

Cultivating Positive Self-Talk

The way individuals talk to themselves during challenging times significantly impacts their resilience. A resilient mindset involves cultivating positive self-talk, fostering self-encouragement and self-compassion.

Mindset shifts for positive self-talk:

- Replacing negative thoughts – actively replacing negative thoughts with positive and empowering affirmations.
- Acknowledging strengths – recognising personal strengths and achievements, even in the midst of challenges.
- Practising self-compassion – treating oneself with kindness and understanding, especially during difficult times.

Mindset as a Protective Factor

A resilient mindset acts as a protective factor against the detrimental effects of stress and adversity. It serves as a buffer, helping individuals bounce back from challenges with greater fortitude.

Mindset shifts for use as a protective factor:

- Reducing stress impact – a resilient mindset reduces the impact of stress, as individuals view challenges as manageable rather than overwhelming.
- Enhancing coping strategies – resilient individuals are more likely to engage in healthy coping strategies, further mitigating the negative effects of adversity.
- Promoting emotional wellbeing – the mindset that resilience is achievable contributes to overall emotional wellbeing, creating a positive cycle of coping and thriving.

The role of mindset in resilience is transformative. By fostering a growth mindset, embracing change, learning from setbacks, building resilience over time, cultivating positive self-talk and recognising mindset as a protective factor, individuals can actively shape their ability to bounce back from adversity. A resilient mindset is not just a response to challenges; it is a proactive approach to life that enhances wellbeing, promotes continuous growth and empowers individuals to navigate the complexities of life with strength and adaptability.

6.2 Cultivating Positive Habits: Building the Foundation for Resilience

Cultivating positive habits is a fundamental aspect of building resilience. These habits act as the building blocks that contribute to mental, emotional and physical wellbeing, creating a sturdy foundation to withstand life's challenges.

Let's take a closer look at the key elements of cultivating positive habits.

Wellness Practices

Physical Wellbeing

Resilience is closely tied to physical health. Positive habits related to physical wellbeing contribute to overall resilience. Regular exercise, a balanced diet and sufficient sleep are essential components.

- Engaging in regular physical activity has been linked to improved mood, reduced stress and enhanced cognitive function. Resilient individuals prioritise regular exercise as part of their routine.
- A well-balanced diet provides the necessary nutrients for both physical and mental health. Resilient individuals make conscious choices about their nutrition, understanding its impact on their overall wellbeing.
- Quality sleep is crucial for resilience. Establishing healthy sleep patterns contributes to emotional stability, cognitive function and the ability to cope with stress.

Mindfulness and Stress Reduction

Cultivating habits related to mindfulness and stress reduction are central to building resilience. These habits promote a calm and focused mind, enabling individuals to navigate challenges more effectively.

- Meditation and mindfulness practices that are incorporated into daily routines foster a present-focused and centred mindset. Resilient individuals often start or end their day with mindful practices.

- Deep-breathing techniques, such as conscious breathing, are simple, yet powerful tools for stress reduction. Resilient individuals develop a habit of incorporating deep breathing exercises during moments of tension or stress.

Connection and Social Support

Nurturing Relationships

Positive habits related to social connections contribute significantly to resilience. Building and maintaining supportive relationships is a key aspect of emotional wellbeing.

- Quality time with loved ones is something resilient individuals prioritise. Positive social interactions contribute to a sense of belonging and emotional support.
- Effective communication ensures individuals can express their needs and feelings. Resilience is often bolstered by the development of communication habits and the ability to share experiences and seek support.
- Active listening, and being fully present in conversations foster deeper connections and strengthen the supportive aspects of relationships. Resilient individuals cultivate the habit of active listening.

Learning and Growth

Continuous Learning

Resilience involves a commitment to continuous learning and personal growth. Cultivating habits that promote intellectual stimulation and curiosity contributes to adaptability.

- Reading and seeking knowledge as an intellectual curiosity broadens perspectives and enhances problem-solving skills. Resilient individuals often have a habit of reading and seeking knowledge.
- Setting and achieving goals creates a sense of purpose. Resilient individuals understand the importance of establishing a routine of setting small, achievable goals that contribute to a larger vision.

- Embracing challenges as opportunities for growth is central to resilience. Rather than avoiding difficulties, resilient individuals approach them as chances to learn and evolve.

Mindful Decision-Making

Incorporating Mindfulness into Daily Life

Mindful decision-making is a habit that contributes to resilience. It involves approaching choices with a clear and present mindset, considering long-term consequences and aligning decisions with personal values.

- Reflective decision-making, and taking the time to consider options, weigh consequences and align choices with personal values, contributes to positive outcomes. Resilient individuals often cultivate the habit of reflective decision-making.
- Adapting to changing circumstances is a key aspect of resilience. Mindful decision-makers are adaptable. They understand that circumstances can change, and decisions may need to be adjusted accordingly.

Gratitude Practices

Cultivating Gratitude

Gratitude practices are powerful habits that contribute to emotional wellbeing and resilience. Regularly acknowledging and appreciating positive aspects of life fosters a positive outlook.

- Gratitude journalling is a common habit among resilient individuals. Writing down things one is grateful for each day cultivates a habit of recognising and appreciating positive aspects of life.
- Expressing thanks, whether through verbal expressions or small gestures, contributes to positive social interactions and strengthens relationships. Resilient individuals actively express gratitude to others.
- Finding joy in small moments contributes to a positive and resilient mindset. Resilient individuals take notice of and savour these moments.

Acts of Kindness

Contributing to Others

Engaging in acts of kindness is a habit that not only benefits others but also enhances one's sense of purpose and community. Resilient individuals actively contribute to the wellbeing of others.

- Random acts of kindness, whether big or small, is a habit that resilient individuals cultivate. These acts create a positive ripple effect, fostering a sense of connection and fulfillment.
- Volunteering regularly is a positive habit that contributes to resilience. It provides individuals with a sense of purpose and allows them to contribute to causes they are passionate about.
- Building a Legacy is a forward-looking mindset that contributes to a sense of purpose and a lasting positive legacy. Resilient individuals often cultivate the habit of considering the impact they want to have on the world.

Cultivating positive habits is integral to building resilience. These habits contribute to overall wellbeing, providing a sturdy foundation for navigating life's challenges. Whether related to physical health, social connections, continuous learning, mindful decision-making, gratitude practices or acts of kindness, positive habits create the proactive and adaptive mindset essential for resilience. By intentionally cultivating these habits, individuals empower themselves to face adversity with strength, adaptability and purpose.

6.3 Developing Problem-Solving Skills: A Cornerstone of Resilience

Effective problem-solving is a cornerstone of resilience, enabling individuals to navigate challenges, adapt to change and bounce back from setbacks. Developing problem-solving skills involves cultivating a mindset that approaches obstacles as opportunities for growth and learning.

Let's take a closer look at the key aspects of developing problem-solving skills.

Analysing Challenges

Breaking Down Challenges

Resilience begins with the ability to analyse challenges methodically. Instead of feeling overwhelmed, individuals with strong problem-solving skills break down complex issues into manageable parts.

- Systems thinking is a holistic approach that allows for a comprehensive understanding. Resilient individuals often employ systems thinking, considering the interconnectedness of different aspects of a challenge.
- Identifying core issues within a challenge is part of developing problem-solving skills. This involves distinguishing between symptoms and root causes.

Setting Realistic Goals

Breaking Down Larger Goals

Resilient individuals set realistic and achievable goals, understanding that progress is often incremental. This habit involves breaking down larger objectives into smaller, actionable steps.

- Creating a roadmap is one way to develop problem-solving skills to achieve goals. This involves planning and organising steps in a logical sequence.
- Monitoring progress by regularly assessing achievements and making necessary adjustments are integral aspects of effective problem-solving. Resilient individuals actively monitor their progress toward goals.

Flexibility and Adaptability

Embracing Change

Resilience is closely tied to the ability to embrace change. Individuals with strong problem-solving skills understand that flexibility and adaptability are key components of overcoming challenges.

- Adapting strategies based on feedback and changing circumstances is key to developing problem-solving skills. Resilient individuals view adaptability as a strength.
- Learning from experience redefines problem-solving capacity. Resilient individuals reflect on past challenges, analysing what worked and what didn't, and adjusting their approach accordingly.

Critical Thinking

Evaluating Options

Critical thinking is at the core of effective problem-solving. Resilient individuals evaluate various options, considering potential outcomes and consequences before making decisions.

- Considering multiple perspectives is a key component of problem-solving. Resilient individuals seek diverse viewpoints to gain a comprehensive understanding of a situation.
- Making informed decisions based on available information is part of critical thinking. Resilient individuals prioritise gathering relevant data before taking action.

Resourcefulness

Creative Problem-Solving

Resilient individuals often display resourcefulness in their problem-solving approach. This involves thinking creatively and finding innovative solutions to challenges.

- Thinking outside the box involves exploring unconventional approaches ad novel ideas. Resilient individuals consider novel ideas and think outside the box.
- Utilising available resources is a form of resourcefulness. Resilient individuals leverage their skills, knowledge and networks to address challenges effectively.

Learning from Setbacks

AIterative Problem-Solving

Developing problem-solving skills is an iterative process that includes learning from setbacks. Resilient individuals view setbacks not as failures but as opportunities for refinement and growth.

- Adapting strategies involves being open to trying different approaches when faced with setbacks. Resilient individuals adapt their problem-solving strategies.
- Resilience through reflecting on setbacks is a habit that contributes to resilience. Resilient individuals actively engage in self-reflection, extracting valuable lessons from challenges.

Maintaining Emotional Regulation

Calm and Composed Decision-Making

Emotional regulation is a crucial aspect of effective problem-solving. Resilient individuals maintain a calm and composed state, allowing for clearer decision-making during challenging situations.

- Mindfulness in decision-making utilises a clear and present mindset when problem-solving. Resilient individuals integrate mindfulness into their decision-making process.
- Managing stress and anxiety bolsters resilience. Individuals with strong problem-solving skills develop healthy coping mechanisms to navigate emotional challenges.

Developing problem-solving skills is integral to building resilience. It involves cultivating a mindset that approaches challenges as opportunities for growth, embraces change and leverages creative and critical thinking. Resilient individuals actively analyse challenges, set realistic goals, demonstrate flexibility, engage in critical thinking, exhibit resourcefulness, learn from setbacks and maintain emotional regulation. These problem-solving skills contribute to a proactive and adaptive approach to life, empowering individuals to navigate complexities with resilience and effectiveness. By honing these skills, individuals not only enhance their ability to overcome obstacles but also foster a mindset that promotes continuous growth and learning.

6.4 Building Emotional Intelligence: Navigating Challenges with Insight

Building emotional intelligence is a key aspect of resilience, enabling individuals to navigate challenges with self-awareness, self-regulation, empathy and effective interpersonal relationships. Emotional intelligence contributes to a deeper understanding of emotions, fostering adaptive responses to stress and adversity. There are several key elements in building emotional intelligence:

Recognising and Understanding Emotions

Emotional Awareness

Building emotional intelligence begins with cultivating emotional awareness. Resilient individuals actively recognise and understand their emotions, and develop a nuanced awareness of how emotions influence their thoughts and behaviours.

- Mindful observation involves non-judgmental awareness, allowing for a more accurate understanding of emotional experiences. Individuals building emotional intelligence practise mindful observation of their emotions.
- Identifying triggers involves being attuned to situations or circumstances that may evoke specific emotional responses. Resilient individuals with emotional intelligence can identify emotional triggers.

Acceptance of Emotions

Validating Emotions

A critical aspect of emotional intelligence is the acceptance and validation of emotions. Resilient individuals understand that all emotions, even uncomfortable ones, are valid and provide valuable information about their internal state.

- Cultivating emotional resilience involves accepting a wide range of emotions. Resilient individuals embrace emotions without judgement, allowing for a more adaptive response to challenges.

- Avoiding emotional suppression allows resilient individuals to express emotions in healthy ways. Emotional intelligence involves avoiding the suppression of emotions and prevents the buildup of internal stress.

Emotional Regulation

Healthy Coping Mechanisms

Building emotional intelligence includes the development of healthy coping mechanisms for regulating emotions. Resilient individuals engage in activities that promote emotional wellbeing and prevent negative emotional states from escalating.

- Creative expression is a part of emotional regulation. Resilient individuals may use art, writing or other forms of expression to channel and process their emotions.
- Physical activity is a common strategy for emotional regulation. Exercise has been shown to have positive effects on mood and stress reduction.

Empathy and Compassion

Understanding Others

Emotional intelligence extends to understanding and empathising with the emotions of others. Resilient individuals develop strong interpersonal skills, fostering supportive and positive relationships.

- Active listening is part of having empathy. Resilient individuals listen attentively to others, seeking to understand their perspectives and emotions without judgement.
- Providing support to others is a key factor in possessing emotional intelligence. Resilient individuals offer compassion and assistance to those going through difficult times.

Emotional Intelligence in Interpersonal Relationships

Conflict Resolution

Building emotional intelligence contributes to effective conflict resolution. Resilient individuals navigate conflicts with emotional intelligence, understanding their own emotions and those of others involved.

- Effective communication is enhanced in emotionally intelligent individuals. Resilient individuals express themselves clearly and assertively, while being attuned to the emotional nuances of communication.
- Building positive relationships is a direct result of developing emotional intelligence. Resilient individuals create connections based on mutual understanding and support.

Emotional Intelligence in Decision-Making

Balancing Emotions and Logic

In decision-making, emotional intelligence involves finding a balance between emotions and logic. Resilient individuals make decisions that consider both the emotional and rational aspects of a situation.

- Mindful decision-making is evident in those who are building emotional intelligence. Resilient individuals approach decisions with a clear understanding of their emotional state and its potential impact.
- Adaptability in decision-making is possible when one possesses emotional intelligence. Resilient individuals are open to adjusting their decisions based on new information or changing circumstances.

Fostering Emotional Intelligence in Others

Promoting Emotional Literacy

Resilient individuals actively contribute to fostering emotional intelligence in others. This involves promoting emotional literacy and creating environments that value emotional expression and understanding.

- Teaching emotional regulation is possible for those who are building emotional intelligence. Resilient individuals may mentor others by sharing strategies for developing healthy coping mechanisms.
- Encouraging open communication allows emotional intelligence to thrive. Resilient individuals create spaces where individuals feel safe expressing their emotions.

Building emotional intelligence is a transformative process that enhances resilience. It involves recognising and understanding emotions, accepting them without judgement, regulating emotional responses, empathising with others and applying emotional intelligence to interpersonal relationships and decision-making. Resilient individuals actively cultivate emotional intelligence as a skill that not only contributes to their own wellbeing but also positively influences the dynamics of their relationships and the broader community. By prioritising emotional intelligence, individuals strengthen their capacity to navigate challenges with insight, adaptability and a profound understanding of the human experience.

6.5 Fostering a Sense of Purpose: The Heartbeat of Resilience

Fostering a sense of purpose is a powerful component of resilience, providing individuals with a guiding light and a reason to persevere through challenges. A clear sense of purpose not only acts as a source of motivation but also contributes to mental and emotional fortitude.

Let's take a closer look at the key aspects of fostering a sense of purpose.

Defining Personal Values and Beliefs

Clarifying Core Values

Fostering a sense of purpose begins with a deep exploration of personal values and beliefs. Resilient individuals take the time to clarify what matters most to them, creating a foundation for meaningful purpose.

- Reflecting on one's core beliefs indicates a strong sense of purpose. This introspective process allows for a deeper understanding of one's guiding principles.

- Aligning actions with values creates a sense of authenticity and coherence in the pursuit of purpose. Resilient individuals align their actions and decisions with their core values.

Setting Meaningful Goals

Connecting Goals to Purpose

A sense of purpose is often linked to meaningful goals. Resilient individuals set goals that resonate with their values and contribute to a larger sense of purpose in their lives.

- Long-term visions are required to foster a sense of purpose. Resilient individuals establish goals that extend beyond immediate challenges, contributing to a sense of direction.
- Prioritising impactful goals is essential. Resilient individuals prioritise goals that have a positive impact, not only on their lives but also on the lives of others and the community.

Contributing to Something Larger Than Oneself

Social and Community Connection

A robust sense of purpose often involves contributing to something larger than oneself. Resilient individuals actively seek ways to connect with and contribute to their communities.

- Community engagement contributes to fostering a sense of purpose. Resilient individuals participate in activities that contribute positively to the wellbeing of the community.
- Social impact can be achieved through small acts of kindness or larger initiatives. Resilient individuals consider the broader impact of their actions and seek to make a positive difference.

Finding Meaning in Adversity

Turning Challenges into Opportunities

A resilient sense of purpose allows individuals to find meaning in adversity. Resilient individuals view challenges as opportunities for growth, learning and a deeper understanding of their purpose.

- Refining purpose through setbacks can help foster a sense of purpose. Resilient individuals use challenges as moments for reflection and adjustment.
- Learning from difficult experiences is essential. Resilient individuals use difficult experiences as lessons that contribute to a more nuanced and resilient sense of purpose.

Cultivating Intrinsic Motivation

Connecting Passion to Purpose

Fostering a sense of purpose involves connecting intrinsic motivations and passions to overarching life goals. Resilient individuals find joy and fulfillment in pursuing what truly matters to them.

- Intrinsic rewards are derived when individuals align actions with purpose. Resilient individuals seek intrinsic rewards that then become a satisfying and powerful motivator during challenging times.
- Passion-driven resilience helps cultivate a sense of purpose. Individuals are more likely to persevere through difficulties when fueled by a deep passion for their chosen path.

Adapting Purpose Over Time

Flexibility in Purpose

Fostering a sense of purpose is not a static process, but evolves over time. Resilient individuals recognise the need for flexibility and adaptation in their sense of purpose.

- Life transitions may necessitate adjustments to one's sense of purpose. Resilient individuals adapt their goals and aspirations to align with evolving values and priorities.

- Continual reflection can help foster a sense of purpose. Resilient individuals regularly reassess their goals, ensuring their sense of purpose remains relevant and meaningful.

Connecting Purpose to Wellbeing

Holistic Wellbeing

A resilient sense of purpose contributes to holistic wellbeing. Resilient individuals experience a deeper sense of satisfaction and contentment, knowing their actions are aligned with a purpose that extends beyond individual fulfillment.

- Emotional resilience is enhanced by fostering a sense of purpose. Individuals are better equipped to navigate emotional challenges when they are anchored in a purpose that provides meaning.
- Psychological wellbeing is often experienced by resilient individuals at a higher level. A clear sense of purpose contributes to a positive mindset and a more optimistic outlook on life.

Fostering a sense of purpose is the heartbeat of resilience, providing individuals with the motivation and direction to navigate challenges with determination. By clarifying values, setting meaningful goals, contributing to the community, finding meaning in adversity, cultivating intrinsic motivation, adapting purpose over time and connecting purpose to overall wellbeing, individuals can strengthen their resilience. A robust sense of purpose not only empowers individuals to endure difficulties but also enhances their ability to find purpose and meaning in the journey of life.

6.6 Mindfulness and Present-Moment Awareness: Anchors in Resilience

Mindfulness and present-moment awareness are foundational practices that contribute significantly to resilience. They involve cultivating a heightened state of awareness and presence, allowing individuals to navigate challenges with clarity, focus and a sense of calm.

Let's take a closer look at the key aspects of mindfulness and present-moment awareness.

Understanding Mindfulness

Present-Moment Focus

Mindfulness is the practice of bringing one's attention to the present moment. Resilient individuals actively cultivate present-moment awareness, allowing them to engage fully in their experiences without being overly reactive or overwhelmed.

- Observing thoughts and emotions without judgement is part of mindfulness. Resilient individuals approach their internal experiences with a sense of curiosity and acceptance.
- Anchoring to the breath is a common mindfulness technique. This practice fosters a centred and calm state, even amid challenging circumstances.

Benefits of Mindfulness in Resilience

Emotional Regulation

Mindfulness plays a crucial role in emotional regulation, which is a key aspect of resilience. Resilient individuals leverage mindfulness to manage and respond to emotions effectively.

- Reduction in physiological stress responses can be a result of mindfulness practice. Resilient individuals use these practices to mitigate the impact of stress on their overall wellbeing.
- Enhancing emotional intelligence can be a result of mindfulness practice. Through mindfulness, resilient individuals gain a deeper understanding of their emotions and the emotions of others.

Cultivating Present-Moment Awareness

Grounding in the Now

Present-moment awareness involves grounding oneself in the current experience. Resilient individuals actively cultivate this awareness, avoiding unnecessary worry about the future or lingering in past regrets.

- Sensory perception is heightened by present-moment awareness. Resilient individuals notice details in their environment, fostering a deeper connection to the present.
- Non-attachment to thoughts is practised by mindful individuals. Resilience is enhanced as individuals recognise that thoughts are transient and do not define their reality.

Mindfulness in Action

Applying Mindfulness to Challenges

Mindfulness is not confined to formal meditation but can be applied actively in daily life. Resilient individuals use mindfulness in real time to navigate challenges with a calm and focused mindset.

- Mindful decision-making is used by resilient individuals. They make choices with a clear awareness of the present moment, considering the immediate context and long-term consequences.
- Conflict resolution is more effective with mindfulness practice. When faced with conflict, resilient individuals bring a calm and present awareness to the situation, fostering clearer communication and understanding.

Mindful Breathing and Stress Reduction

Breath as an Anchor

Mindful breathing is a powerful tool for stress reduction. Resilient individuals use their breath as an anchor, allowing them to return to the present moment and centre themselves during stressful situations.

- Calming the sympathetic nervous system, which is responsible for the body's stress response, is helped by mindful breathing. This physiological shift enhances resilience in the face of adversity.
- Creating space for response is enhanced through mindfulness practices. Resilient individuals use mindful breathing to help gain the ability to respond thoughtfully, rather than react impulsively to stressors.

Mindfulness Practices for Resilience

Regular Meditation Practice

Resilient individuals often incorporate regular meditation into their routines. Meditation serves as a dedicated time for mindfulness, allowing individuals to develop and strengthen their present-moment awareness.

- Body scan meditation is a mindfulness practice that involves systematically bringing attention to different parts of the body. Resilient individuals use this practice for relaxation and self-awareness.
- Loving-kindness meditation involves cultivating feelings of love and compassion, not only for oneself but also for others. Resilient individuals use loving-kindness meditation to foster a positive and empathetic mindset.

Mindfulness as a Lifelong Skill

Continual Practice

Mindfulness is viewed as a lifelong skill by resilient individuals. It is not a one-time solution but a continual practice that evolves and deepens over time.

- Integration of mindfulness into daily life enhances the individual's ability to stay present and composed amid life's fluctuations. Resilient individuals integrate mindfulness into various aspects of their daily lives.
- Adapting to change is fostered by mindfulness. Through the practice of mindfulness, resilient individuals become more adept at navigating change with grace and an open-minded perspective.

Mindfulness and present-moment awareness serve as anchors in resilience, providing individuals with a heightened state of awareness and a centred presence. By embracing mindfulness, individuals can regulate their emotions, navigate challenges with clarity and cultivate a deeper connection to the present moment. This practice becomes not just a tool for stress reduction but a way of life that enhances resilience and empowers individuals to face life's uncertainties with equanimity and strength.

By understanding the dynamic nature of resilience, cultivating positive habits, developing problem-solving skills, building emotional intelligence, fostering a sense of purpose and incorporating mindfulness into daily routines, individuals can empower themselves to face life's challenges with strength and adaptability. Resilience is not just a trait but a way of life, shaping responses to adversity and contributing to long-term wellbeing. Resilience is embraced as a skill that can be cultivated and strengthened, leading to a more fulfilling and purpose-driven life.

Chapter Seven

Addressing Trauma Triggers and Relapse Prevention

Trauma recovery is a nuanced journey that involves not only unpacking the impact of past traumatic experiences but also navigating the present challenges that can trigger distressing memories and emotions.

Chapter 7 delves into the critical aspects of addressing trauma triggers and implementing relapse prevention strategies, providing individuals with the tools and insights necessary for sustained healing and resilience.

7.1 Understanding Trauma Triggers: Navigating the Complex Terrain

The journey of trauma recovery is fraught with challenges, and a critical aspect of this process involves understanding and managing trauma triggers. Trauma triggers are stimuli or situations that elicit strong emotional and psychological reactions, reminiscent of past traumatic experiences. In this exploration, we delve into the nuances of trauma triggers, understanding their origins, categories and the profound impact they can have on individuals navigating the path of healing.

The Complexity of Trauma Triggers

Trauma triggers are not uniform; they manifest in diverse forms, arising from a complex interplay of psychological, emotional and environmental factors. Understanding these triggers requires a nuanced exploration that acknowledges the unique nature of each individual's traumatic experiences.

Origins of Trauma Triggers

Trauma triggers often stem from associations formed during the traumatic event. These associations link specific stimuli, such as sights, sounds or even smells, to the emotional and physiological responses experienced during the trauma. For instance, a loud noise resembling a gunshot might trigger intense anxiety in someone who has survived a violent incident.

These triggers are not solely external; internal factors, including thoughts, emotions or bodily sensations, can also serve as powerful triggers. Understanding the interplay of internal and external triggers is fundamental to crafting effective coping strategies.

The Neurobiology of Trauma Triggers

The brain's response to trauma is a key element in understanding triggers. The amygdala, a region associated with processing emotions, particularly fear, plays a pivotal role. During a traumatic event, the amygdala becomes hyperactive, creating strong associations between the traumatic experience and the stimuli present at the time.

In the aftermath, encountering similar stimuli can activate the amygdala, triggering a cascade of responses, including the release of stress hormones. This physiological response can lead to a heightened state of arousal, anxiety or even a flashback to the traumatic event.

Categories of Trauma Triggers

Trauma triggers manifest across various domains of human experience. Categorising triggers helps individuals and therapists comprehend their diverse nature, facilitating a targeted approach to trigger management.

Environmental Triggers

Environmental triggers encompass stimuli present in the individual's surroundings. These might include specific locations, objects or even weather conditions. For instance, a survivor of a car accident may find it challenging to drive or be near busy traffic without experiencing heightened anxiety.

Sensory Triggers

Sensory triggers involve stimuli that engage the senses, such as touch, smell or taste. A survivor of a physical assault might be triggered by a touch that resembles the touch experienced during the trauma. Similarly, specific scents or tastes can evoke powerful memories associated with the traumatic event.

Interpersonal Triggers

Interpersonal triggers are linked to relationships and social interactions. These triggers can emerge when the dynamics of a current relationship resemble those of the traumatic past. For example, someone who experienced betrayal might be triggered by situations that involve perceived betrayal in their present relationships.

Internal Triggers

Internal triggers are rooted in an individual's internal states, including thoughts, emotions and bodily sensations. Internal triggers might include feelings of shame, guilt or specific thought patterns associated with the trauma. Understanding and navigating internal triggers is crucial for comprehensive trigger management.

Recognising the Impact of Trauma Triggers

The impact of trauma triggers extends beyond the immediate emotional and physiological responses. They can disrupt daily functioning, strain relationships and contribute to a pervasive sense of anxiety and hypervigilance.

Disruption of Daily Functioning

Trauma triggers can disrupt various aspects of daily life. Routine activities, such as going to work, grocery shopping or even sleeping, can become challenging when specific triggers are present. This disruption not only affects the individual's well-being but also contributes to a sense of frustration and helplessness.

Strain on Relationships

Interpersonal triggers, in particular, can strain relationships. The inability to navigate social interactions without being triggered may lead to social withdrawal, isolation or conflict within relationships. Friends and family members, though often well-intentioned, may find it challenging to understand the profound impact triggers can have on an individual's emotional landscape.

Persistent Anxiety and Hypervigilance

The constant threat of encountering triggers can contribute to persistent anxiety and hypervigilance. Individuals may develop heightened alertness, always anticipating potential triggers and adjusting their behaviour to avoid distress. This state of hyperarousal can be exhausting and further exacerbate the emotional toll of trauma.

Therapeutic Exploration of Trauma Triggers

The therapeutic journey involves a collaborative exploration of trauma triggers between individuals and their therapists. This exploration is multifaceted, involving the identification of triggers, understanding their origins and developing effective strategies for managing and mitigating their impact.

Trigger Mapping as a Therapeutic Tool

Trigger mapping is a valuable therapeutic tool in understanding the intricate web of trauma triggers. This process involves collaboratively creating a visual representation of triggers, their associated emotions and the circumstances in which they arise. Trigger maps provide a comprehensive overview, offering insights into patterns and potential areas for intervention.

Journalling for Trigger Awareness

Encouraging individuals to maintain trigger journals fosters ongoing self-awareness. Journalling allows individuals to document trigger incidents, the emotions they elicit and any thoughts associated with the triggers. Over time, this practice contributes to a deeper understanding of the nature of the triggers and the factors that exacerbate or alleviate their impact.

Mindfulness Practices for Present-Moment Awareness

Mindfulness practices are integral to the therapeutic exploration of trauma triggers. Mindfulness involves cultivating present-moment awareness without judgement. Through mindfulness, individuals learn to observe their thoughts, emotions and bodily sensations, enhancing their capacity to recognise triggers as they arise. Mindfulness also provides a valuable tool for managing the distress that triggers can evoke.

Trauma Triggers in the Context of Identity and Self-Concept

Trauma has a profound impact on an individual's sense of self. Trauma triggers, often intertwined with one's identity, can evoke complex emotions related to self-worth, shame and identity.

Identity Disruption and Trauma Triggers

Traumatic experiences can disrupt an individual's sense of identity. Triggering situations may challenge an individual's narrative about themselves, contributing to feelings of inadequacy or self-doubt. Therapeutic exploration involves not only understanding the triggers themselves, but also addressing the broader implications for an individual's self-concept.

Shame and Trauma Triggers

Shame is a common emotional response to trauma triggers, particularly triggers associated with interpersonal trauma. Individuals may experience shame about their reactions to triggers, believing that they should be able to cope more effectively. Shame can become a barrier to seeking support and engaging in the therapeutic process. Therapists work delicately to navigate the terrain of shame, fostering an environment of compassion and acceptance.

Trauma Triggers and the Therapeutic Relationship

The therapeutic relationship plays a pivotal role in the exploration and management of trauma triggers. Trust and collaboration between the individual and therapist form the foundation for effective trigger intervention.

Trust as a Catalyst for Trigger Exploration

Establishing trust is a gradual process in the therapeutic relationship. Trust allows individuals to disclose and explore their triggers openly. Therapists cultivate an environment where individuals feel safe to share their trigger experiences without fear of judgement or invalidation.

Collaborative Intervention Strategies

Interventions for trauma triggers are collaborative endeavours. Therapists work closely with individuals to develop personalised strategies for managing triggers. This collaboration empowers individuals to take an active role in their trigger management, fostering a sense of agency and control.

Trauma Triggers and the Journey of Healing

Understanding trauma triggers is not only about managing distress but also about creating a roadmap for healing and resilience. The journey involves not just the identification and avoidance of triggers but a transformational process that allows individuals to reclaim agency over their lives.

Empowerment Through Trigger Management

Effective trigger management is an empowering process. As individuals learn to navigate triggers, they gain a sense of mastery over their emotional responses. This empowerment extends beyond trigger-specific incidents, influencing how individuals approach challenges in other areas of their lives.

Trauma-Informed Strategies for Long-Term Resilience

Trauma-informed strategies for trigger management go beyond immediate coping mechanisms. Therapists guide individuals in developing a comprehensive toolkit for long-term resilience. This may involve exposure-based approaches, cognitive restructuring and the cultivation of healthy coping mechanisms.

Navigating Trauma Triggers as a Transformative Journey

Understanding trauma triggers is an intricate process that requires compassion, insight and collaboration. In the therapeutic space, individuals embark on a transformative journey where triggers cease to be insurmountable obstacles and become opportunities for growth and healing. Through this understanding, the path to resilience and recovery unfolds, allowing individuals to reclaim their narratives and forge ahead into a future marked by empowerment and self-discovery.

7.2 Developing Trigger Awareness: A Crucial Step in Trauma Recovery

In the intricate landscape of trauma recovery, the development of trigger awareness emerges as a pivotal step. Triggers, stimuli that evoke memories and emotions associated with past traumatic experiences, can significantly impact an individual's wellbeing. Developing awareness involves a comprehensive exploration of triggers, from their origins to their manifestation, and equips individuals with the tools to navigate their emotional landscape. This journey of self-discovery is a collaborative effort between individuals and their therapists, fostering an understanding that lays the groundwork for effective trigger management.

Unravelling the Layers of Trigger Awareness

Understanding triggers requires delving into the multifaceted layers that contribute to their existence. It involves unravelling the cognitive, emotional and physiological dimensions intertwined with the traumatic experience. This process is not only about recognising external stimuli, but also about deciphering internal cues and thought patterns that serve as potent triggers.

The Cognitive Dimension of Triggers

Cognitions, encompassing thoughts and beliefs, play a fundamental role in triggering emotional responses. These cognitions often operate on a subconscious level, influencing how individuals interpret and react to the world around them. For example, an individual who has experienced a traumatic event involving betrayal may develop automatic thoughts such as "I can't trust anyone" or "People will always let me down". Identifying and unravelling these cognitive patterns are key aspects of trigger awareness.

The Emotional Landscape of Triggers

Emotions act as powerful indicators of triggers. The emotional responses elicited by certain situations or stimuli provide clues to the underlying triggers at play. Understanding the intricate web of emotions involves recognising not only the overt reactions, such as fear or sadness, but also the subtle nuances that may signify the presence of triggers. Emotional awareness forms a bridge between the conscious and subconscious realms, allowing individuals to navigate the complexities of their internal world.

The Physiological Response to Triggers

The body often holds the residue of trauma, manifesting in physiological responses to triggers. These responses can range from an increased heart rate and shallow breathing to more pronounced reactions like panic attacks or dissociation. Developing awareness of these physiological cues involves attuning to the body's signals and discerning patterns that indicate the activation of trauma-related responses. The interplay between the cognitive, emotional and physiological dimensions creates a comprehensive understanding of triggers.

Therapeutic Techniques for Unveiling Triggers

In the therapeutic space, unveiling triggers is a delicate and collaborative process. Therapists employ various techniques to guide individuals in developing awareness, fostering a nuanced understanding of their triggers.

Trigger Mapping: A Visual Exploration

Trigger mapping, a visual representation of triggers and their associated elements, serves as a powerful therapeutic tool. In collaboration with their therapists, individuals create maps that depict specific triggers, the emotions they evoke and the circumstances surrounding their occurrence. This visual exploration not only provides a tangible record but also facilitates a deeper understanding of the intricate connections between triggers and their contextual cues.

Journalling: Capturing the Narrative of Triggers

Journalling becomes a reflective space for individuals to capture the narrative of their triggers. Regular journal entries document trigger incidents, the emotions experienced and any thoughts that arise. Over time, this narrative becomes a valuable resource for individuals and therapists alike, offering insights into patterns, the evolution of the triggers and the effectiveness of coping mechanisms.

Mindfulness Practices: Cultivating Present-Moment Awareness

Mindfulness practices serve as a cornerstone in developing trigger awareness. Mindfulness involves cultivating present-moment awareness without judgement. By focusing attention on thoughts, emotions and bodily sensations as they arise, individuals enhance their capacity to recognise triggers in real-time. Mindfulness also fosters a non-reactive stance, allowing individuals to observe triggers without being engulfed by their intensity.

Cultivating Self-Reflection and Insight

The journey of trigger awareness is deeply intertwined with self-reflection. Individuals embark on a process of introspection, cultivating the ability to reflect on their thoughts, emotions and behaviours. This self-reflective practice contributes to a heightened awareness of internal states and the factors that may precede or accompany trigger incidents.

The Role of Therapeutic Self-Reflection

Therapists guide individuals in therapeutic self-reflection, creating a space for them to explore their experiences in a supported environment. This process involves reflecting on trigger incidents, identifying the associated emotions and discerning patterns in cognitive and emotional responses. Therapeutic self-reflection is not about self-blame but rather a compassionate inquiry into one's internal landscape.

Developing Insight through Narrative Exploration

Narrative exploration becomes a vehicle for developing insight into triggers. Therapists work with individuals to delve into the stories they tell themselves about their triggers. These narratives may include beliefs about safety, trust and self-worth. By unpacking these narratives, individuals gain insight into the layers of meaning attached to their triggers, paving the way to reframing these narratives.

The Interplay of Triggers with Identity and Beliefs

Triggers are intricately interwoven with an individual's sense of identity and beliefs about themselves and the world. Recognising this interplay forms a crucial component of trigger awareness.

Triggers as Mirrors Reflecting Identity

Triggers often act as mirrors reflecting aspects of an individual's identity. They illuminate core beliefs about oneself, others and the world. For instance, a trigger related to a past rejection might be intricately linked to beliefs about one's lovability or worthiness. Acknowledging triggers as reflections of identity opens avenues for exploration and transformation.

The Dance Between Triggers and Self-Concept

The dance between triggers and self-concept is dynamic. Triggers can reinforce negative self-perceptions and contribute to a distorted self-concept. Conversely, as individuals develop awareness and challenge these negative beliefs, the dance transforms. Therapists guide individuals in navigating this intricate dance, supporting them in reshaping their self-concept in the light of newfound awareness.

The Therapeutic Relationship as a Catalyst for Awareness

The therapeutic relationship serves as a catalyst for the development of trigger awareness. Trust and collaboration within this relationship create a safe space for individuals to explore the depths of their triggers without fear of judgement or invalidation.

Trust as the Foundation of Awareness

Establishing trust between individuals and their therapists is foundational. Trust provides the necessary scaffolding for individuals to share their most vulnerable experiences, including the intricacies of their triggers. Therapists nurture an environment where individuals feel heard, understood and supported, fostering a sense of safety conducive to awareness development.

Collaboration in Unveiling Triggers

The therapeutic relationship thrives on collaboration. Therapists and individuals collaborate in the exploration of triggers, combining their insights and perspectives. This collaborative approach empowers individuals to actively participate in their healing journey, fostering a sense of agency and control over their trigger awareness.

The Role of Community and Peer Support

Beyond the therapeutic relationship, community and peer support contribute significantly to the development of trigger awareness. Engaging with a supportive community provides individuals with additional perspectives, shared experiences and a sense of belonging.

Shared Narratives in Community Spaces

Community spaces, whether in-person or online, offer platforms for individuals to share their narratives. The act of articulating one's triggers and hearing others' experiences creates a sense of validation and normalises the varied responses to trauma. Shared narratives contribute to a broader understanding of triggers and offer a diverse range of coping strategies.

Peer Support in Navigating Awareness

Peer support becomes a valuable resource in the journey of trigger awareness. Individuals navigating similar challenges can offer insights, practical tips and empathetic understanding. Peer support groups, facilitated by trained professionals or as informal networks, create spaces where individuals feel seen and heard in their quest for trigger awareness.

Strategies for Navigating Trigger Awareness Challenges

While the journey of developing trigger awareness is transformative, it is not without challenges. Individuals may encounter resistance, emotional intensity or feelings of overwhelm. Therapists play a crucial role in guiding individuals through these challenges.

Navigating Resistance with Compassion

Resistance may arise as individuals confront painful or uncomfortable aspects of their triggers. Therapists approach resistance with compassion, recognising it as a natural response to the vulnerability inherent in the awareness process. Gentle exploration and the gradual pace of self-discovery are essential components of navigating resistance.

Managing Emotional Intensity

The emotional intensity that accompanies trigger awareness can be overwhelming. Therapists provide tools for emotional regulation, such as grounding techniques and mindfulness practices. Acknowledging and validating the intensity of emotions is part of the therapeutic process, fostering a supportive environment for individuals to navigate these emotional landscapes.

Gradual Exposure and Building Resilience

Gradual exposure to triggers, conducted in a controlled and therapeutic setting, forms part of the awareness process. Therapists guide individuals through carefully planned exposures, allowing them to build resilience and emotional regulation. The objective is not to overwhelm but to empower individuals to face triggers with increasing levels of mastery.

Integrating Trigger Awareness into Daily Life

The true essence of trigger awareness lies in its integration into daily life. This involves the translation of insights gained in therapy into practical strategies that individuals can implement independently.

Daily Practices for Sustaining Awareness

Individuals are encouraged to establish daily practices that sustain trigger awareness. This may include brief moments of mindfulness, regular journalling or engaging in self-reflective exercises. Consistency in these practices contributes to the ongoing development of awareness.

Applying Trigger Management Techniques

The insights gained through trigger awareness translate into practical trigger management techniques. Individuals develop a repertoire of strategies, including cognitive restructuring, grounding techniques and mindfulness, which they can apply when triggers arise. The goal is to move from reactive responses to triggers to a more intentional and empowered approach.

The Ongoing Journey: Beyond Trigger Awareness

While trigger awareness is a profound milestone, the journey of trauma recovery extends beyond this awareness. It is a continuous process of growth, self-discovery and resilience-building. Therapists guide individuals in recognising the potential for ongoing development and transformation.

Navigating Evolving Triggers

As individuals grow and evolve, so too may their triggers. Life transitions, new experiences and personal growth can introduce new elements that trigger memories or emotions. Navigating evolving triggers involves adapting awareness strategies and continuing the collaborative work with therapists.

Harnessing Trigger Awareness for Empowerment

Trigger awareness becomes a tool for empowerment. Individuals harness their awareness to make informed choices, set boundaries and engage in activities that align with their values. The process becomes a journey of self-empowerment, where individuals actively shape their lives per their newfound understanding.

Trigger Awareness as a Transformative Journey

Developing trigger awareness is a transformative journey that encapsulates the intricate process of self-discovery, healing and empowerment. It involves unravelling the layers of triggers, understanding their cognitive, emotional and physiological dimensions and integrating this awareness into daily life. In the therapeutic space, individuals find support, guidance and a collaborative environment that fosters their journey toward holistic wellbeing. Trigger awareness is not just a milestone, it is a dynamic process that propels individuals toward a future marked by resilience, agency and a profound connection with their own narratives.

7.3 Trauma-Informed Strategies for Trigger Management: Navigating the Path to Healing

In the intricate tapestry of trauma recovery, the effective management of triggers stands as a pivotal component. Trauma-informed strategies for trigger management go beyond mere coping mechanisms; they encompass a comprehensive approach that acknowledges the profound impact of trauma on individuals' lives. This exploration delves into trauma-informed strategies, unveiling a roadmap for navigating triggers with sensitivity, understanding and a commitment to fostering resilience.

Understanding Trauma-Informed Care

At the heart of trauma-informed trigger management is the concept of trauma-informed care. This paradigm shift in care delivery recognises the prevalence of trauma and emphasises creating environments that are safe, empowering and cognisant of the unique needs of trauma survivors.

The Core Principles of Trauma-Informed Care

Trauma-informed care is grounded in several core principles.

- *Safety*: prioritising physical and emotional safety creates a foundation for healing. This involves creating environments where individuals feel secure and respected.
- *Trustworthiness and transparency*: building trust is paramount. Transparent communication and clear expectations contribute to a sense of predictability and reliability.
- *Peer support and mutual help*: the recognition of the healing power of supportive relationships, including peer support, fosters a sense of community and shared understanding.
- *Collaboration and mutuality*: collaboration between individuals and their support network, including therapists, creates a sense of shared responsibility in the healing journey.
- *Empowerment, voice and choice*: providing individuals with a sense of agency and the ability to make choices in their care promotes empowerment and autonomy.

The Role of Trauma-Informed Care in Trigger Management

Trauma-informed care is seamlessly integrated into trauma trigger management. It guides therapists and individuals in navigating triggers with sensitivity and understanding, recognising that triggers are not just isolated incidents but manifestations of deeper trauma-related experiences.

Holistic Approaches to Trigger Management

Trauma-informed strategies for trigger management adopt a holistic perspective, addressing the interconnected aspects of individuals' lives.

Addressing Biological Aspects: Regulation and Grounding Techniques

The physiological responses to triggers are central to trauma recovery. Strategies that focus on regulation, such as grounding techniques, help individuals navigate heightened arousal states. These techniques may include mindfulness exercises, deep breathing or sensory grounding activities. By anchoring individuals in the present moment, these practices foster a sense of safety and stability.

Psychological Approaches: Cognitive Restructuring and Reframing

Cognitive restructuring involves identifying and challenging negative thought patterns associated with triggers. Through therapeutic interventions, individuals learn to reframe distorted cognitions, replacing them with more adaptive and balanced beliefs. This cognitive shift contributes to a change in emotional responses to triggers, promoting a more resilient mindset.

Emotional Regulation: Dialectical Behaviour Therapy (DBT) and Mindfulness

Dialectical Behaviour Therapy (DBT) and mindfulness practices play a crucial role in emotional regulation. DBT, with its emphasis on distress tolerance and emotion regulation, equips individuals with practical skills to manage intense emotions triggered by past trauma. Mindfulness, woven into DBT and as a standalone practice, enhances present-moment awareness, allowing individuals to observe and regulate their emotional responses to triggers.

Social and Relational Approaches: Building Supportive Networks

Social support is a cornerstone of trauma recovery. Trauma-informed trigger management involves recognising the importance of supportive relationships. Therapists collaborate with individuals to identify and nurture supportive networks, fostering a sense of belonging and reducing the impact of triggers through shared experiences and understanding.

Creating Safe Spaces: Physical and Emotional Safety

Central to trauma-informed trigger management is the creation of safe spaces. These spaces extend beyond physical environments to encompass emotional safety within therapeutic relationships and daily interactions.

Physical Safety: Establishing Boundaries

Creating physically safe spaces involves establishing clear boundaries. In therapy, therapists work collaboratively with individuals to set and communicate boundaries that ensure a sense of physical safety. This may include discussing comfort levels with touch, pacing of sessions and creating a non-threatening environment.

Emotional Safety: Trust and Therapeutic Alliance

Emotional safety is nurtured through the development of trust within the therapeutic alliance. Therapists prioritise building a trusting relationship, recognising that this trust forms the bedrock for exploring triggers. Transparent communication, empathy and attunement to the emotional needs of individuals contribute to the emotional safety required for effective trigger management.

Trauma-Informed Strategies for Specific Triggers

Trauma triggers are diverse, and trauma-informed strategies recognise the need for specificity in their management. Different triggers may require tailored approaches to ensure effective intervention.

Triggers Associated with Interpersonal Trauma: Establishing Trust

Individuals who have experienced interpersonal trauma may grapple with triggers related to trust and safety in relationships. Trauma-informed care involves gradually building trust within therapeutic relationships and providing opportunities for individuals to express their fears and concerns. Establishing a sense of control and choice within the therapeutic process is integral to managing interpersonal triggers.

Triggers Linked to Shame and Guilt: Compassionate Exploration

Triggers associated with shame and guilt necessitate a compassionate exploration of these complex emotions. Trauma-informed strategies involve acknowledging and validating these feelings while challenging distorted self-perceptions. Therapists guide individuals in reframing shame-inducing thoughts, fostering self-compassion and separating the self from the actions or circumstances that led to the trauma.

Triggers Manifesting as Flashbacks: Grounding Techniques

Flashbacks – vivid and distressing recollections of traumatic events – can be profoundly challenging. Trauma-informed care incorporates grounding techniques to anchor individuals in the present during flashbacks. Grounding may involve engaging the senses, such as holding onto a comforting object or focusing on the physical sensations in the body. This redirection of attention helps individuals regain a connection with the present, mitigating the intensity of flashbacks.

Triggers in Daily Environments: Gradual Exposure and Desensitization

Triggers embedded in daily environments, such as specific sounds or locations, may be addressed through gradual exposure. This trauma-informed strategy involves systematically and safely exposing individuals to elements of their triggers. Therapists collaborate with individuals to create a hierarchy of exposure, allowing for a progressive and controlled approach to desensitisation.

Trauma-Informed Strategies for Long-Term Resilience

Beyond immediate trigger management, trauma-informed strategies aim at cultivating long-term resilience. This involves equipping individuals with a toolkit of skills and practices that contribute to ongoing wellbeing.

Empowerment Through Education: Understanding Triggers

Knowledge is empowering. Trauma-informed care includes psychoeducation about triggers, helping individuals understand the neurobiological and psychological aspects of their reactions. This knowledge fosters self-awareness and reduces the unpredictability surrounding triggers, contributing to a more empowered approach to trigger management.

Skill-Building for Coping and Resilience

Trauma-informed strategies prioritise skill-building for coping and resilience. This may involve learning and practising mindfulness, developing effective communication skills and honing problem-solving abilities. The acquisition of these skills empowers individuals to navigate challenges beyond therapy sessions, fostering a sense of mastery over their lives.

Narrative Empowerment: Reframing Trauma Stories

Narrative empowerment involves reframing trauma stories. Trauma-informed care recognises the impact of the narratives individuals construct around their traumatic experiences. Therapists collaborate with individuals to explore alternative narratives that emphasise resilience, growth and strengths. This reframing contributes to a sense of agency in shaping one's life story.

A Trauma-Informed Journey Toward Healing

Trauma-informed strategies for trigger management form an integral part of the journey toward healing and resilience. Grounded in principles of safety, trust and empowerment, these strategies navigate the complexities of triggers with sensitivity and understanding. By addressing the biological, psychological and social dimensions of triggers, trauma-informed care offers a holistic approach that recognises the multifaceted impact of trauma. The ultimate goal is not just the management of triggers but the cultivation of a resilient and empowered individual who is capable of navigating life's challenges with newfound strength and understanding.

7.4 Relapse Prevention Strategies in Trauma Recovery: Navigating the Path to Sustained Healing

The journey of trauma recovery is marked by its complexities and the risk of relapse is a significant consideration in this process. Relapse in trauma recovery refers to the recurrence or intensification of symptoms after a period of improvement. Relapse prevention strategies play a crucial role in fostering sustained healing, recognising that setbacks can be part of the nonlinear nature of recovery. This exploration delves into the multifaceted strategies designed to prevent and navigate relapses in the context of trauma recovery.

Understanding the Dynamics of Relapse in Trauma Recovery

Before delving into prevention strategies, it's essential to understand the dynamics of relapse in trauma recovery. Relapses are not indicative of failure; rather, they highlight the intricate nature of healing from trauma.

Triggers and Vulnerability Factors

Triggers, as discussed earlier, can play a pivotal role in relapses. These triggers can be diverse, ranging from environmental cues to interpersonal dynamics. Understanding individual vulnerability factors is equally crucial. These may include co-occurring mental health conditions, life stressors, or a lack of robust coping mechanisms.

The Nonlinear Nature of Trauma Recovery

Trauma recovery is rarely a linear process. It involves peaks and valleys, progress and setbacks. Acknowledging the nonlinear nature of recovery is foundational to understanding relapse. Individuals may make substantial progress and then encounter challenges that trigger a resurgence of symptoms. Relapse prevention strategies are designed to navigate these fluctuations and minimise the impact of setbacks.

Holistic Approaches to Relapse Prevention

Relapse prevention in trauma recovery requires a holistic approach that addresses various dimensions of an individual's life.

Therapeutic Continuity: Sustaining the Therapeutic Alliance

Maintaining a strong therapeutic alliance is central to relapse prevention. Consistency in therapeutic sessions provides individuals with a stable and supportive space. Therapists collaborate with individuals to anticipate potential triggers, develop coping strategies and continually reassess treatment goals. This ongoing dialogue fosters adaptability in the therapeutic process.

Building Coping Repertoire: Skill Development

One of the primary contributors to relapse prevention is the development of a robust coping repertoire. Therapists work with individuals to identify and enhance coping skills that are effective for their unique needs. This may include cognitive-behavioural strategies, mindfulness practices and emotion regulation techniques. The goal is to equip individuals with a diverse toolkit for managing challenges.

Holistic Self-Care: Nurturing the Body and Mind

Self-care is a cornerstone of relapse prevention. This involves nurturing the body and mind through practices that promote overall wellbeing. Therapists guide individuals in developing self-care routines encompassing physical health, emotional regulation and activities that bring joy and relaxation. Holistic self-care contributes to resilience in the face of stressors.

Identifying and Managing Triggers in Real Time

Proactive identification and management of triggers form a key component of relapse prevention. Therapists collaborate with individuals to create awareness around their triggers and develop strategies for real-time intervention.

Trigger Identification: Anticipating Challenges

Therapists work with individuals to identify potential triggers, considering internal and external factors. This involves exploring past triggers, understanding the context in which they arose, and anticipating challenges that may emerge in the future. By developing this awareness, individuals are better prepared to recognise and respond to triggers.

Real-Time Intervention: Coping Strategies

In the moment of a trigger, effective coping strategies are vital. Therapists assist individuals in designing personalised interventions that can be implemented when triggers occur. These may include grounding techniques, self-soothing practices or reaching out to a support network. Real-time interventions empower individuals to navigate triggers actively.

Strengthening Resilience Through Mindset Shifts

A resilient mindset is a powerful asset in relapse prevention. Therapists collaborate with individuals to cultivate mindset shifts that contribute to long-term resilience.

Positive Psychology Practices: Focusing on Strengths

Positive psychology practices involve shifting the focus from pathology to strengths. Therapists work with individuals to identify and cultivate their strengths, fostering a positive self-concept. This shift contributes to resilience by reframing challenges as opportunities for growth.

Empowerment Through Narrative: Reframing Stories

Narrative empowerment involves reframing one's life story. Therapists guide individuals in constructing narratives that emphasise resilience and agency. This process of narrative reframing contributes to a sense of empowerment, reducing the impact of past traumas on individuals' identities.

Community and Peer Support in Relapse Prevention

Beyond individual efforts, community and peer support play crucial roles in relapse prevention. Therapists encourage individuals to build and leverage supportive networks.

Community Engagement: Finding a Sense of Belonging

Engaging with communities that share similar experiences provides a sense of belonging. Therapists assist individuals in finding and participating in support groups, community activities or online forums where shared narratives foster understanding and validation.

Peer Mentorship: Learning from Shared Experiences

Peer mentorship offers a unique form of support. Individuals who have navigated similar challenges can provide insights, practical advice and empathetic understanding. Therapists facilitate connections between individuals in different stages of recovery, creating opportunities for shared learning.

Continuous Evaluation and Adaptation of Treatment Plans

Relapse prevention is an ongoing process that requires continuous evaluation and adaptation of treatment plans. Therapists and individuals collaborate to monitor progress, reassess goals and make necessary adjustments.

Regular Treatment Reviews: Assessing Progress

Regular treatment reviews involve assessing the effectiveness of current strategies and identifying areas for improvement. Therapists and individuals engage in open discussions about challenges, successes and evolving needs. This collaborative process ensures that the treatment plan remains aligned with the individual's goals.

Flexibility in Approaches: Adapting to Changing Needs

Flexibility in treatment approaches is essential. Individuals may encounter new triggers or life circumstances that require adjustments to coping strategies. Therapists work collaboratively to adapt interventions, ensuring they remain relevant and effective in addressing evolving challenges.

Recognition and Management of Co-occurring Conditions

Co-occurring mental health conditions can contribute to relapse risk. Relapse prevention involves the recognition and management of these conditions in tandem with trauma-focused interventions.

Integrated Treatment Plans: Addressing Dual Challenges

Integrated treatment plans consider the interconnected nature of trauma and co-occurring conditions. Therapists collaborate with individuals and, when necessary, with other healthcare professionals to create comprehensive plans that address both trauma and concurrent mental health challenges.

Psychoeducation on Co-occurring Conditions

Psychoeducation plays a vital role in relapse prevention. Individuals gain an understanding of how co-occurring conditions may interact with trauma symptoms. This knowledge enhances self-awareness and informs proactive strategies for managing both trauma and other mental health aspects.

Cultivating a Forward-Looking Perspective

Relapse prevention is not only about managing the present but also about cultivating a forward-looking perspective. Therapists assist individuals in envisioning and working towards a future marked by sustained wellbeing.

Goal-Setting and Future Planning

Goal-setting becomes a collaborative process between therapists and individuals. These goals may encompass various domains, including relationships, career and personal development. Setting and working towards achievable goals contribute to a sense of purpose and motivation for the future.

Embracing the Process: Patience and Self-Compassion

Relapse prevention involves embracing the process of recovery with patience and self-compassion. Therapists guide individuals in recognising that setbacks are not indicative of failure but rather opportunities for learning and growth. Developing resilience involves navigating challenges with a compassionate and forward-looking perspective.

Family Involvement in Relapse Prevention

Family dynamics can significantly impact relapse risk. Therapists work with individuals and their families to create a supportive and understanding environment.

Psychoeducation for Families: Understanding Trauma

Family members gain insights into the effects of trauma through psychoeducation. Understanding the nuances of trauma contributes to empathy and informed support. Therapists facilitate family sessions to address questions and concerns and develop strategies to contribute to a supportive home environment.

Open Communication and Boundaries

Open communication is vital in families affected by trauma. Therapists guide individuals and their families in establishing healthy communication patterns. This involves setting boundaries, expressing needs and fostering an environment where individuals feel heard and understood.

Collaborative Crisis Planning: A Contingency Approach

In the event of a crisis or relapse, having a collaborative crisis plan in place is essential. Therapists and individuals work together to develop a contingency approach that outlines steps to be taken in case of setbacks.

Crisis Intervention Strategies: Immediate Support

Crisis intervention strategies involve immediate support in the face of relapse. Therapists collaboratively develop crisis plans that may include emergency contacts, coping strategies and steps to regain a sense of safety. This proactive approach ensures that individuals have a roadmap to navigate crises.

Post-Crisis Evaluation: Learning and Growth

Post-crisis evaluations contribute to the learning and growth process. Therapists engage in reflective discussions with individuals, exploring the factors that led to the crisis and identifying strategies to mitigate future risks. This collaborative evaluation reinforces resilience and adaptability in the face of setbacks.

Empowering Individuals in the Face of Relapse

Relapse prevention in trauma recovery is an empowering process that involves a collaborative and multifaceted approach. By addressing triggers, cultivating resilience and involving support networks, individuals are equipped with the tools to navigate challenges effectively. The journey of sustained healing is marked not only by the absence of relapses but also by the ability to learn, adapt, and continue forward with newfound strength and understanding. Therapists play a crucial role in guiding individuals through this process, fostering a sense of agency and resilience that extends beyond the therapeutic space.

7.5 Empowering Individuals for Long-Term Resilience

Addressing trauma triggers and implementing relapse prevention strategies is a collaborative endeavour that empowers individuals to build resilience for the long term. Therapists play a vital role in instilling a sense of agency and self-efficacy, fostering the belief that individuals can navigate challenges and maintain progress in their trauma recovery journey.

Building a Resilience Mindset

A resilience mindset involves cultivating the belief that challenges can be navigated, setbacks can be overcome, and growth is an inherent part of the recovery process. Therapists support individuals in:

- developing cognitive flexibility, adapting to changing circumstances and viewing challenges from multiple perspectives
- recognising and reinforcing positive adaptive behaviours, contributeing to the development of a resilient mindset.

Integration of Self-Care Practices

Self-care practices are integral to maintaining emotional and psychological wellbeing. Therapists collaborate with individuals to:

- customise self-care plans to individual preferences, ensuring that practices are sustainable and enjoyable
- promote consistency when it comes to engagement in self-care activities as a way of contributing to emotional regulation and stress management.

Embracing the Learning Process

Trauma recovery is a continuous learning process. Therapists guide individuals in:

- reflective practices, such as journalling or mindfulness, to support ongoing self-awareness and learning
- skills development, particularly when it comes to learning and honing coping skills and resilience-building strategies, to contribute to increased self-efficacy.

7.6 A Roadmap to Lasting Recovery

Addressing trauma triggers and implementing relapse prevention strategies is a dynamic and ongoing process that aligns with each individual's unique journey of healing. By understanding the nature of triggers, developing awareness and employing trauma-informed strategies, individuals gain a toolkit to navigate challenges effectively.

Relapse prevention, as an integral part of trauma recovery, involves averting crises and reinforcing positive behavioural patterns and building long-term resilience. As guides and collaborators, therapists play a central role in empowering individuals to take charge of their recovery, navigate setbacks with resilience and embrace the transformative journey toward lasting healing. In the next chapter, we will delve into additional dimensions of trauma recovery, exploring avenues for growth, self-discovery and the cultivation of a meaningful and fulfilling life beyond the shadows of trauma.

Chapter Eight

❦

Moving Forward and Thriving

The journey of trauma recovery extends beyond the process of healing; it encompasses the vision of moving forward and not merely surviving but thriving.

Chapter 8 explores the essential elements and strategies that contribute to this transformative phase. Moving forward and thriving after trauma is not just about overcoming adversity; it involves cultivating a life rich in purpose, resilience, and meaningful connections. In this chapter, we delve into the nuanced aspects of this forward trajectory, emphasising empowerment, growth and the attainment of a fulfilling and thriving existence.

8.1 Shaping a New Narrative: From Victim to Survivor to Thriver

The process of recovering from trauma involves a fundamental shift in the narrative individuals construct about their experiences. This transformation is not merely a linguistic exercise but a profound redefinition of one's identity, a journey from victimhood to survivorship, and ultimately, to a state of thriving. This chapter's pivotal theme — the shaping of a new narrative — explores the nuanced dynamics involved in transitioning from a victim defined by traumatic experiences to a survivor who has navigated adversity and, ultimately, to a thriver who actively shapes a future filled with purpose and resilience.

Redefining Identity

Embracing the Survivor Identity

The initial phase of this transformation involves embracing the identity of a survivor. Therapists play a crucial role in guiding individuals through this shift, helping them recognise the strength and resilience that allowed them to endure and overcome the traumatic event. The survivor identity is not just a label but a reclamation of agency — an acknowledgment that, despite the impact of trauma, individuals possess an inherent capacity to overcome adversity.

Recognising Personal Agency

Therapists employ various therapeutic modalities to facilitate the recognition of personal agency. Cognitive-behavioral approaches help individuals challenge and reframe disempowering beliefs about themselves. Narrative therapy techniques encourage the exploration of personal strengths and the identification of moments of agency, fostering a sense of control over one's narrative.

Empowerment Through Narrative Reframing

Reconstructing the Trauma Narrative

Narrative reframing becomes a powerful tool in empowering individuals to shape a new narrative. This involves not erasing the traumatic event but reconstructing the narrative around it. Therapists guide individuals to explore alternative interpretations, emphasising resilience, growth and personal strengths. The goal is to create a narrative that transcends victimhood, emphasising the individual's capacity to navigate and learn from adversity.

Positive Psychology Interventions

Positive psychology interventions contribute significantly to this process. Practices such as identifying and utilising personal strengths, cultivating gratitude and fostering a positive mindset become integral. These interventions shift the focus from the trauma as a defining factor to the individual as an active agent in their own story, capable of deriving meaning and purpose from their experiences.

Transitioning to the Thriver Identity

Beyond Surviving: Embracing Thriving

The transition from survivor to thriver marks a profound evolution. Thriving is not just about overcoming the aftermath of trauma but actively pursuing a life filled with meaning, connection and personal fulfillment. Therapists collaborate with individuals to explore aspirations, values and goals, guiding them towards a future-oriented mindset.

Building a Future-Oriented Mindset

Therapists engage in goal-setting exercises with individuals, encouraging them to articulate their aspirations and map out steps toward realising those goals. This forward-looking perspective is instrumental in breaking free from the constraints of the past. Individuals learn to view challenges not as insurmountable obstacles but as opportunities for growth and development.

A Transformative Journey

Shaping a new narrative — from victim to survivor to thriver — is a transformative journey guided by therapeutic collaboration. Therapists provide the scaffolding for individuals to reconstruct their narratives, emphasising resilience, agency and potential for growth. The journey is not linear, and individuals may revisit different aspects of their narrative at various stages of the recovery process. However, the overarching goal is clear — to empower individuals not just to survive their traumas but to thrive despite them.

This theme sets the tone for the broader exploration of post-traumatic growth. It acknowledges the profound impact of trauma while asserting that individuals possess an innate capacity for resilience and thriving. As individuals shape their new narratives, they embark on a journey of self-discovery and empowerment, ultimately realising that the narrative they construct about their past has the power to shape their future.

8.2 Cultivating Resilience for Long-Term Wellbeing

Cultivating resilience is a cornerstone of long-term wellbeing for individuals on the journey towards trauma recovery. Resilience goes beyond mere survival; it entails bouncing back from adversity, adapting positively to challenges and building the psychological and emotional strength needed to navigate life's complexities. The significance of resilience for sustained wellbeing is profound. Here, we explore the dynamic process of building and nurturing resilience over time.

Resilience as a Dynamic Process

Understanding Resilience

Resilience is not a fixed trait but a dynamic process that can be nurtured and strengthened. Therapists engage individuals in a collaborative exploration of resilience, helping them recognise that it is not a predetermined quality but an adaptive response to life's adversities. This understanding forms the foundation for intentional efforts to enhance resilience throughout the trauma recovery journey.

Therapeutic Approaches to Enhance Resilience

Therapists employ evidence-based approaches to enhance resilience. Cognitive-behavioural therapy (CBT) helps individuals identify and reframe negative thought patterns that may hinder resilience. Mindfulness-based interventions, such as Mindfulness-Based Stress Reduction (MBSR), contribute to resilience by fostering present-moment awareness and emotional regulation. By integrating these approaches, therapists empower individuals to develop a resilient mindset.

Integrating Positive Psychology Practices

Positive Psychology and Resilience

Positive psychology practices play a pivotal role in the cultivation of resilience. Therapists introduce individuals to exercises that focus on strengths, gratitude and positive reframing. By consciously directing attention towards positive aspects of life, individuals can begin to shift their perspective from a deficit-oriented mindset to one that appreciates and amplifies their inherent strengths.

Strengths-Based Approaches

Identifying and leveraging personal strengths is a key component of positive psychology interventions. Therapists collaboratively work with individuals to explore and recognise their unique strengths. By emphasising strengths, individuals develop a reservoir of internal resources that can be drawn upon during challenging times, contributing to greater resilience.

Navigating Relationships and Building Social Support

Rebuilding Trust in Relationships

Trauma often fractures trust in interpersonal relationships. Therapists guide individuals in rebuilding trust, emphasising effective communication, setting healthy boundaries and establishing realistic expectations. By fostering a sense of safety in relationships, individuals can draw on their social support networks as a source of strength.

The Role of Social Support Networks

Thriving after trauma is inherently connected to the cultivation of a robust support network. Therapists assist individuals in identifying and nurturing supportive relationships, whether within family, friendships or community. A reliable support network acts as a buffer during challenging times, enhancing overall resilience.

Romantic Relationships and Intimacy

Navigating romantic relationships after trauma requires a nuanced approach. Therapists guide communication, trust-building and integrating intimacy into the healing process. Individuals learn to approach relationships with a sense of self-awareness and the tools to foster healthy connections.

Pursuing Meaning and Purpose

Meaning-Making as a Transformative Process

Thriving after trauma does not just involve recovering from the past, but also finding meaning in the present and future. Therapists assist individuals to make meaning, helping them identify personal values, set meaningful goals and discover a sense of purpose that transcends the traumatic experience.

Career and Educational Pursuits

Occupational and educational pursuits play a significant role in the pursuit of meaning and purpose. Therapists collaborate with individuals to explore career paths aligned with their passions and strengths. This might involve career counselling, skills development or educational opportunities that contribute to a sense of fulfillment and purpose.

Contribution to Community and Society

Thriving extends beyond personal fulfillment to contributing meaningfully to the broader community and society. Therapists guide individuals in exploring avenues for community engagement, volunteering or advocacy work. This provides a sense of purpose and also reinforces the idea that one's experiences can be harnessed for positive change.

Building Resilience for a Thriving Future

Cultivating resilience is not a one-time endeavour but an ongoing process that intertwines with the broader trajectory of trauma recovery. The exploration of resilience sets the stage for a future-oriented mindset. Individuals learn to navigate relationships, pursue meaning and build a support network that fortifies their wellbeing. Therapists play a pivotal role in this process, guiding individuals to harness their innate resilience and empowering them to not just endure, but thrive in the face of adversity. As resilience becomes an integral part of their psychological toolkit, individuals are better equipped to face life's challenges with strength, adaptability and purpose.

8.3 Navigating Relationships and Building Social Support

Navigating relationships and building a robust social support network is a crucial component of the trauma recovery journey. This section explores how therapists guide individuals in rebuilding trust, fostering healthy relationships and establishing a network of support that becomes instrumental in the process of thriving.

Rebuilding Trust in Relationships

Understanding the Impact of Trauma on Trust

Trauma often leaves individuals with fractured trust in relationships. Betrayal, loss or violation experienced during the traumatic event can significantly impact the ability to trust others. Therapists acknowledge this impact, providing a safe space for individuals to express their concerns and fears related to trust.

Therapeutic Strategies for Rebuilding Trust

Therapists employ strategies such as trust-building exercises and psychoeducation on trust dynamics. Cognitive-behavioural approaches help individuals identify and challenge negative beliefs about trust that may have developed as a result of the trauma. By addressing these beliefs, therapists lay the groundwork for rebuilding trust in both interpersonal and professional relationships.

The Role of Social Support Networks

Identifying and Nurturing Supportive Relationships

The cultivation of a robust social support network is central to thriving after trauma. Therapists work collaboratively with individuals to identify existing supportive relationships and explore opportunities to nurture new connections. This process involves recognising the qualities of healthy relationships and establishing boundaries that contribute to a sense of safety and support.

Family Dynamics and Support

Family relationships play a pivotal role in the recovery process. Therapists conduct family sessions, providing psychoeducation on the effects of trauma and offering a platform for open communication. Individuals and their families explore ways to strengthen familial bonds, ensuring that the family becomes a source of support rather than a potential stressor.

The Significance of Friendships

Friendships are often a cornerstone of social support. Therapists guide individuals to identify friends who can offer understanding, empathy and encouragement. Building or rekindling friendships becomes an essential component of the recovery process, providing individuals with a network beyond familial connections.

Community and Group Support

In addition to individual relationships, therapists explore community and group support options. Group therapy sessions, community organisations or support groups become spaces where individuals can connect with others who have experienced similar challenges. The shared understanding within these groups fosters a sense of belonging and reduces feelings of isolation.

Romantic Relationships and Intimacy

Navigating Intimacy After Trauma

Trauma can deeply impact an individual's ability to engage in and navigate intimate relationships. Therapists approach this aspect with sensitivity, recognising that the restoration of trust and the reintegration of intimacy into one's life is a gradual process. Open communication, consent and establishing emotional safety become focal points of therapeutic interventions.

Communication Strategies for Couples

For individuals in romantic relationships, therapists facilitate communication strategies. Couples engage in dialogue about their needs, expectations and concerns. Therapists guide partners in understanding how trauma may affect the dynamics of the relationship, fostering empathy and mutual support.

Rebuilding Intimacy: A Gradual Process

Rebuilding intimacy is approached as a gradual process. Therapists work with individuals and couples to set realistic goals, establish boundaries and identify activities that contribute to emotional and physical intimacy. This phased approach allows individuals to regain a sense of control over their experiences.

Fostering Resilient Relationships

In the intricate landscape of trauma recovery, navigating relationships and building social support is akin to weaving a safety net for individuals. When we place a spotlight on this vital aspect, we recognise that resilient relationships are the foundation of the process of thriving. Therapists act as guides, helping individuals rebuild trust, foster connections and create a support network that becomes a cornerstone of their journey towards a fulfilling and meaningful life. As individuals learn to navigate relationships with a newfound understanding and resilience, they not only enhance their wellbeing but also contribute to the broader tapestry of connected and thriving communities.

8.4 Pursuing Meaning and Purpose

In the aftermath of trauma, the pursuit of meaning and purpose emerges as a transformative process, steering individuals away from the mere recovery of the past toward a future rich in significance and fulfillment. In this section, we explore meaning-making and purpose-building, highlighting the therapeutic strategies employed to guide individuals on this journey.

Meaning-Making as a Transformative Process

Understanding Meaning-Making

Meaning-making involves the active construction of an understanding or narrative about the significance of one's experiences. Therapists recognise that trauma can shatter existing frameworks of meaning, leaving individuals grappling with existential questions. In therapy, the process of meaning-making is explored as a transformative endeavour, allowing individuals to derive coherence and purpose from their lived experiences.

Therapeutic Approaches to Meaning-Making

Therapists employ various therapeutic modalities to facilitate meaning-making. Narrative therapy encourages individuals to construct a coherent and empowering narrative about their experiences. Existential therapy delves into the exploration of existential themes such as freedom, responsibility, and the search for meaning. By engaging in reflective dialogue, individuals are supported in their quest to derive personal significance from their journey.

Career and Educational Pursuits

Aligning with Personal Values

Career and educational pursuits are integral components of the meaning-making process. Therapists collaborate with individuals to identify personal values and aspirations. This involves exploring career paths that align with an individual's passions and principles. The therapeutic space becomes a canvas where career goals are articulated, and strategies for pursuing these goals are developed.

Skill Development and Education

Skill development and education play a pivotal role in the pursuit of meaning and purpose. Therapists guide individuals in acquiring the skills necessary for their chosen paths, whether through formal education, vocational training, or skill-building activities. This enhances employability and also contributes to competence and mastery.

The Role of Occupational Therapy

Occupational therapy becomes a valuable tool in the pursuit of purposeful activities. Therapists collaborate with individuals to identify meaningful and fulfilling occupations. This may involve engaging in hobbies, volunteer work or the exploration of entrepreneurial ventures that align with an individual's sense of purpose.

Contribution to Community and Society

From Self-Discovery to Contribution

Thriving after trauma extends beyond personal fulfillment to contributing meaningfully to the broader community and society. Therapists guide individuals in exploring avenues for community engagement, volunteering or advocacy work. This process involves recognising that one's experiences can be harnessed for positive change, transforming personal adversity into a catalyst for societal impact.

Advocacy and Social Justice

Therapists may facilitate conversations around advocacy and social justice, empowering individuals to use their voices to address systemic issues related to their trauma. This advocacy work becomes a source of purpose, as well as a means of effecting change on a broader scale.

Community Integration

The integration into community life becomes a therapeutic goal. Therapists collaborate with individuals to identify community resources, support networks, and opportunities for social engagement. This process is marked by a shift from isolation to active participation, reinforcing the idea that individuals are not only receivers of support but contributors to the wellbeing of their communities.

Building a Meaningful Future

This section underscores the profound impact of pursuing meaning and purpose in the trajectory of trauma recovery. Therapists play a guiding role in this transformative process, assisting individuals in constructing narratives that transcend the trauma and fostering a sense of purpose that extends far beyond survival. As individuals pursue meaningful careers, engage in purposeful activities and contribute to their communities, they not only reclaim their agency but also become architects of a future rich in significance and fulfillment. In the quest for meaning and purpose, the therapeutic journey becomes a powerful exploration of self-discovery and is testament to the resilience inherent in the human spirit.

8.5 Holistic Wellbeing: Mind, Body and Spirit

The pursuit of holistic wellbeing transcends the conventional boundaries of mental health to encompass the interconnected realms of mind, body and spirit. Therapists embark on a comprehensive journey with individuals, recognising that true thriving after trauma involves nurturing all aspects of one's being. This section explores therapeutic strategies that guide individuals toward holistic wellbeing, fostering vitality, resilience and interconnectedness.

Integrative Approaches to Health

Understanding the Mind-Body Connection

Holistic wellbeing begins with an understanding of the mind-body connection. Therapists introduce individuals to the intricate interplay between mental and physical health, emphasising that the state of one profoundly influences the other. This foundational knowledge forms the basis for integrative approaches to health that go beyond traditional mental health interventions.

Mindfulness Practices for Mental Wellbeing

Mindfulness practices are instrumental in nurturing mental wellbeing. Therapists introduce individuals to mindfulness meditation, a practice that cultivates present-moment awareness. Mindfulness not only reduces symptoms of anxiety and depression but also enhances overall mental resilience, fostering clarity and calmness.

Incorporating Physical Activity

Physical activity is integrated into the therapeutic process as a means of promoting mental and emotional wellbeing. Therapists collaborate with individuals to develop personalised fitness routines, recognising that regular exercise not only contributes to physical health but also releases endorphins (neurotransmitters that elevate mood).

Mindfulness and Present-Moment Awareness

The Power of Present Moment-Awareness

Mindfulness and present-moment awareness emerge as transformative tools in the pursuit of holistic wellbeing. Therapists guide individuals in cultivating the ability to be fully present in the moment, free from the burdens of past trauma or anxieties about the future. This practice reduces stress and fosters acceptance and appreciation for life as it unfolds.

Mindful Breathing Exercises

Therapists introduce mindful breathing exercises as a simple yet powerful technique for anchoring oneself in the present moment. By focusing on the breath, individuals learn to regulate their emotions, reduce anxiety and cultivate heightened awareness. This practice becomes a cornerstone of holistic well-being, fostering a connection between the mind and the breath.

Resolving Unfinished Business: Closure and Forgiveness

The Process of Closure

Holistic wellbeing involves addressing unfinished business from the past. Therapists facilitate the process of closure by encouraging individuals to explore and, when appropriate, confront elements of their history that may be hindering their progress. This may involve revisiting specific memories, addressing unexpressed emotions or finding symbolic ways to mark the end of a chapter.

The Complex Nature of Forgiveness

Forgiveness emerges as a nuanced aspect of holistic wellbeing. Therapists recognise that forgiveness is a personal journey and not a universal prescription. Individuals explore the possibility of forgiveness as a means of releasing themselves from the emotional weight of resentment. This process is conducted with care, acknowledging the complexity of forgiving in the context of trauma.

Integration of Spirituality and Transcendence

Spiritual Resilience

For some individuals, spirituality becomes a source of strength and resilience. Therapists support individuals in exploring their spiritual beliefs or practices, integrating them into their healing journey. This may involve finding solace in religious teachings, connecting with nature or exploring existential questions that contribute to transcendence.

Transcending Victimhood Through Spiritual Growth

Spiritual growth offers a pathway to transcend the identity of a victim. Therapists guide individuals in connecting with a deeper sense of self and purpose, fostering spiritual resilience that transcends the limitations of trauma. This spiritual integration contributes to an overarching sense of thriving.

Holistic Self-Care Practices

The Importance of Self-Care

Holistic wellbeing is sustained through intentional self-care practices. Therapists collaborate with individuals to develop personalised self-care routines that address mental, physical and emotional needs. This may involve activities including journalling, creative expression or spending time in nature.

Creative Expression as a Therapeutic Outlet

Creative expression becomes a therapeutic outlet for holistic wellbeing. Therapists encourage individuals to explore creative endeavours, such as art, music or writing, as a means of self-discovery and emotional expression. This creative process enhances mental wellbeing and contributes to personal joy and fulfillment.

8.6 Resolving Unfinished Business: Closure and Forgiveness

The process of resolving unfinished business is transformative and a critical step in the journey towards holistic wellbeing after trauma. Therapists play a pivotal role in guiding individuals through the nuanced terrain of closure and forgiveness. This section delves into the therapeutic strategies employed to facilitate closure, the complex nature of forgiveness and the impact these processes have on an individual's path toward resilience and thriving.

The Process of Closure

Acknowledging Unresolved Elements

Closure involves addressing lingering and unresolved elements from the past. Therapists create a safe space for individuals to acknowledge and explore aspects of their history that continue to exert influence on their present emotional landscape. This may include unexpressed emotions, unanswered questions or lingering attachments to traumatic events.

Therapeutic Techniques for Closure

Therapists employ a range of therapeutic techniques to facilitate closure. Cognitive-behavioural approaches help individuals identify and challenge distorted thought patterns related to unresolved elements. Narrative therapy provides a framework for individuals to reconstruct their narratives, emphasising growth, resilience and the emergence of a new chapter in their lives.

Symbolic Acts and Rituals

Symbolic acts and rituals become powerful tools in the closure process. Therapists work with individuals to identify symbolic gestures or rituals that mark the end of a particular chapter. This may involve writing letters, creating art or engaging in activities that symbolise letting go and moving forward. These symbolic acts serve as bridges between the past and the present, facilitating a sense of closure.

The Complex Nature of Forgiveness

Understanding Forgiveness

Forgiveness, a cornerstone of closure, is approached with sensitivity and recognition of its complexity. Therapists guide individuals in understanding that forgiveness is a personal journey and does not necessarily imply reconciliation with those who caused harm. It is an internal process that frees the individual from the burden of resentment and allows for emotional healing.

Therapeutic Dialogue on Forgiveness

Therapists engage individuals in therapeutic dialogue about forgiveness, exploring their beliefs, values and fears associated with this process. Cognitive restructuring is often employed to challenge rigid beliefs about forgiveness and encourage a more nuanced and self-compassionate perspective.

Stages of Forgiveness

Forgiveness is recognised as a multi-stage process. Therapists help individuals navigate these stages, which may include acknowledging the pain, understanding the perspectives of others involved and ultimately arriving at a place of acceptance and release. This phased approach acknowledges the complexity of forgiveness and respects the individual's unique journey.

Forgiveness as a Form of Empowerment

Reclaiming Personal Power

Forgiveness is reframed as a form of empowerment. Therapists guide individuals in recognising that forgiveness does not diminish the impact of the trauma or invalidate their experiences. Instead, it is a reclaiming of personal power — a conscious choice to no longer be defined by the actions of others. This shift in perspective contributes to a sense of agency and resilience.

Self-Forgiveness

The concept of self-forgiveness is explored as an integral part of the forgiveness process. Therapists assist individuals in releasing self-blame and cultivating self-compassion. This internal forgiveness becomes a crucial aspect of healing, allowing individuals to move beyond guilt and shame toward a more compassionate relationship with themselves.

Closure and Forgiveness in the Therapeutic Journey

Tailoring Approaches to Individual Needs

Therapists recognise that closure and forgiveness are highly individualised processes. Approaches are tailored to the unique needs, values and cultural contexts of each individual. Therapeutic interventions are culturally sensitive and acknowledge the diversity of perspectives on closure and forgiveness.

Integrating Closure and Forgiveness in Trauma-Focused Therapies

Closure and forgiveness are integrated into trauma-focused therapeutic modalities. Eye Movement Desensitization and Reprocessing (EMDR), for example, may incorporate elements of closure as individuals process traumatic memories. Cognitive Processing Therapy (CPT) often includes forgiveness work as part of cognitive restructuring.

Continuous Exploration in the Therapeutic Relationship

Closure and forgiveness are viewed as ongoing explorations within the therapeutic relationship. Therapists remain attuned to shifts in an individual's readiness for closure or forgiveness, recognising that these processes may unfold over an extended period. The therapeutic journey becomes a collaborative exploration, allowing individuals the time and space needed for meaningful resolution.

8.7 Integration of Spirituality and Transcendence

The exploration of holistic wellbeing delves into the profound realm of spirituality and transcendence. Recognising that individuals on the path of trauma recovery may seek solace and meaning beyond traditional therapeutic approaches, this section explores the integration of spirituality as a potent resource for resilience and transcendence. Therapists play a pivotal role in guiding individuals on this spiritual journey, fostering an understanding of the self that extends beyond the trauma narrative.

Spiritual Resilience

Recognising Spirituality as a Resource

Spirituality is acknowledged as a resource for resilience in the face of trauma. Therapists engage individuals in conversations about their spiritual beliefs, recognising the diverse ways in which individuals draw strength from their faith, connection with a higher power or existential exploration. This recognition forms the foundation for integrating spirituality into the broader framework of trauma recovery.

Spiritual Narratives in Therapy

Therapists employ narrative therapy techniques to explore spiritual narratives. Individuals are invited to share their spiritual stories, examining how their beliefs have shaped their understanding of trauma and resilience. This narrative exploration provides insights into the individual's coping mechanisms, sources of strength and the role of spirituality in their meaning-making process.

Connecting with Nature and Existential Themes

Nature as a Source of Transcendence

The connection between spirituality and nature is explored as a means of transcendence. Therapists recognise the healing power of nature and guide individuals in reconnecting with the natural world. This may involve ecotherapy or nature-based interventions that provide a space for reflection, contemplation and connection with something larger than oneself.

Exploring Existential Themes

Existential themes, such as the search for meaning and the nature of human existence, are woven into therapeutic discussions. Therapists guide individuals in exploring existential questions, helping them find purpose and significance amid trauma. This existential exploration becomes a pathway to transcendence, offering a broader context for understanding one's place in the universe.

Transcending Victimhood Through Spiritual Growth

Shifting Perspectives on Victimhood

Spiritual growth is presented as a transformative means of transcending the identity of a victim. Therapists facilitate shifts in perspectives, guiding individuals to view their experiences through the lens of spiritual growth. This involves reframing the narrative from one of victimhood to a story of resilience and spiritual evolution.

Rituals and Ceremonies

Rituals and ceremonies become integral components of spiritual growth. Therapists collaborate with individuals to design rituals that mark significant milestones in their spiritual journey. These ceremonies provide a tangible and symbolic way to honour the process of transcendence and celebrate the strength that arises from spiritual resilience.

Empowering Through Spiritual Practices

Personalised Spiritual Practices

Therapists work with individuals to identify and cultivate personalised spiritual practices. This may include prayer, meditation, mindfulness or engagement with religious rituals. These practices are tailored to align with the individual's beliefs and preferences, empowering them to integrate spirituality into their daily lives as a source of strength and grounding.

Spiritual Mentoring and Guidance

For individuals seeking deeper spiritual exploration, therapists may facilitate connections with spiritual mentors or guides. This mentoring provides a supportive space for individuals to deepen their understanding of spiritual principles, receive guidance on their journey and explore ways in which spiritual insights can inform their trauma recovery.

Cultural Sensitivity and Diversity in Spiritual Integration

Recognising Cultural Diversity

The integration of spirituality is approached with cultural sensitivity, recognising the diversity of spiritual beliefs and practices. Therapists engage in open dialogues about cultural and religious backgrounds, ensuring that the integration of spirituality respects individual diversity and does not impose a particular belief system.

Customising Approaches

Approaches to spiritual integration are customised based on the individual's cultural context. Therapists collaborate with individuals to explore ways in which their cultural and spiritual heritage can be integrated into the therapeutic process. This customisation ensures that spiritual integration is a culturally affirming and enriching experience.

8.8 Building a Future-Oriented Mindset

A future-oriented mindset is a key component of thriving after trauma. Therapists play a crucial role in guiding individuals toward a perspective that goes beyond the constraints of past trauma, fostering resilience and purpose. This section delves into therapeutic strategies for building a future-oriented mindset, envisioning a life that transcends the impact of trauma.

The Dynamic Nature of Resilience

Recognising Resilience as a Dynamic Process

Resilience is presented as a dynamic and evolving process. Therapists work with individuals to recognise the resilience inherent in their journey and help them understand that resilience is not a fixed trait but a capacity that can be nurtured and developed. This reframing empowers individuals to see themselves as capable of adapting and growing in the face of challenges.

Therapeutic Techniques for Enhancing Resilience

Therapists employ cognitive-behavioural techniques to enhance resilience. This may involve identifying and challenging negative thought patterns, cultivating self-compassion and developing a proactive mindset. Narrative therapy is utilised to construct empowering narratives that highlight moments of resilience and strength, providing a foundation for a future-oriented mindset.

The Role of Mindset in Overcoming Challenges

Shifting from a Fixed to a Growth Mindset

Individuals are guided in shifting from a fixed mindset, where abilities and outcomes are seen as predetermined, to a growth mindset that embraces the belief in personal development and the capacity for change. Therapists engage in conversations that challenge limiting beliefs, fostering an understanding that challenges are opportunities for growth rather than insurmountable obstacles.

Cognitive Restructuring for Positive Outlook

Cognitive restructuring techniques are employed to facilitate a positive outlook. Therapists help individuals identify and reframe negative thought patterns related to the future. This involves exploring alternative perspectives and envisioning a future not defined by past traumas. The goal is to cultivate a mindset that is open to possibilities and hopeful about the potential for positive change.

Cultivating Positive Habits

Establishing Habits for Wellbeing

Positive habits become a focal point in cultivating a future-oriented mindset. Therapists collaborate with individuals to identify and establish habits that contribute to wellbeing. This may include routines for self-care, exercise, healthy relationships and activities that bring joy. The integration of positive habits reinforces the idea that the future is shaped by intentional actions in the present.

Behavioural Activation Techniques

Behavioural activation techniques are utilised to counteract patterns of avoidance and withdrawal. Therapists assist individuals in developing a schedule of activities that align with their values and goals. This activation of positive behaviours not only contributes to a sense of accomplishment but also lays the groundwork for a future filled with purpose and meaningful engagement.

Developing Problem-Solving Skills

Embracing a Solution-Focused Approach

Problem-solving skills are integral to a future-oriented mindset. Therapists encourage individuals to embrace a solution-focused approach, emphasising the identification of practical steps to address challenges. Solution-focused brief therapy (SFBT) techniques are employed to help individuals set achievable goals and work towards solutions, fostering agency and control over their future.

Cognitive Behavioural Strategies for Problem-Solving

Cognitive-behavioural strategies are incorporated to enhance problem-solving skills. Therapists guide individuals in breaking down problems into manageable components, challenging unhelpful thoughts that may impede problem-solving, and developing adaptive coping strategies. These skills empower individuals to approach challenges with a proactive and solution-oriented mindset.

Building Emotional Intelligence

Recognising and Regulating Emotions

Emotional intelligence is highlighted as a cornerstone of a future-oriented mindset. Therapists assist individuals in recognising and regulating their emotions. This involves mindfulness practices to increase emotional awareness, cognitive strategies to reframe emotional responses and the development of interpersonal skills for effective emotional expression and communication.

Interpersonal Effectiveness Training

Interpersonal effectiveness training is integrated to enhance emotional intelligence in relationships. Therapists guide individuals in developing assertiveness, active listening and conflict-resolution skills. The cultivation of emotional intelligence in relationships contributes to building a support network and fosters positive connections that align with a future-oriented mindset.

Envisioning and Creating a Thriving Future

Building a future-oriented mindset is a dynamic and multifaceted process. Therapists play a central role in guiding individuals toward resilience, a growth mindset, positive habits, effective problem-solving and emotional intelligence. By envisioning and creating a future that transcends the impact of trauma, individuals not only recover but also thrive. The therapeutic journey becomes a transformative process, empowering individuals to embrace the possibilities that lie ahead, armed with a mindset that is hopeful, proactive and resilient. By embracing a future-oriented perspective, individuals not only reclaim their lives but also contribute to the broader narrative of post-traumatic growth and resilience.

8.9 Collaborative Crisis Planning: A Contingency Approach

Collaborative crisis planning is critical as a contingency approach in trauma recovery. Recognising that crises can be potential triggers for relapse, therapists work collaboratively with individuals to develop comprehensive crisis plans that involve not only the individual in recovery but also their support network. This section delves into the strategies employed in collaborative crisis planning, emphasising the proactive and contingency-focused nature of this approach.

Understanding the Nature of Crises in Trauma Recovery

Definition and Recognition

Therapists engage individuals in discussions that help recognise the diverse nature of crises, ranging from emotional distress to external stressors. Understanding the potential triggers for crises becomes a fundamental step in developing a collaborative crisis plan.

Proactive Anticipation

Therapists encourage a proactive stance toward crises by fostering anticipation. By identifying potential stressors and triggers, individuals can work with their support network to create strategies that mitigate the impact of crises. This anticipatory approach shifts the focus from reactive responses to proactive planning.

The Role of Collaboration in Crisis Planning

Involving the Support Network

Collaborative crisis planning centres on the active involvement of the individual's support network. Therapists facilitate discussions that include family members, friends or any identified sources of support. This collaborative approach ensures that the crisis plan is comprehensive, drawing on the strengths and resources of the entire support system.

Shared Decision-Making

Therapists promote shared decision-making within the collaborative crisis planning process. This involves empowering individuals to express their preferences, needs and coping strategies during a crisis. Engaging in shared decision-making fosters a sense of agency and control, contributing to a more personalised and effective crisis plan.

Developing a Comprehensive Crisis Plan

Individualised Components

Crisis plans are tailored to the individual's unique needs and experiences. Therapists work with individuals to identify specific triggers, warning signs and coping mechanisms that are effective for them. This individualisation ensures that the crisis plan is a dynamic and responsive tool that aligns with the individual's recovery journey.

Inclusion of Coping Strategies

The crisis plan includes a repertoire of coping strategies. Therapists collaborate with individuals to identify coping mechanisms that have proven effective in the past and introduce new strategies when necessary. This may involve incorporating mindfulness techniques, grounding exercises or specific activities that promote emotional regulation.

Crisis Identification and Response

Recognising Warning Signs

A crucial aspect of collaborative crisis planning is the recognition of warning signs. Therapists guide individuals and their support network in identifying early indicators that a crisis may be imminent. This heightened awareness enables a prompt and targeted response, preventing the escalation of the crisis.

Response Protocols

Collaborative crisis plans outline clear response protocols. Therapists work with individuals to establish steps to be taken by the individual in recovery and their support network. This may involve specific communication strategies, designated crisis contacts and emergency resources. Response protocols are designed to be practical, actionable and accessible in times of distress.

Integration of Technology and Resources

Utilising Technology

Technology is integrated into collaborative crisis planning as a tool for immediate support. Therapists explore the use of mobile apps, crisis helplines or virtual support networks that can be accessed during a crisis. The integration of technology ensures that individuals have readily available resources at their fingertips.

Emergency Contacts and Resources

Therapists assist individuals in compiling a list of emergency contacts and resources. This may include mental health professionals, crisis helplines, community organisations or friends and family members. The crisis plan provides clear information on how to access these resources during a crisis, fostering a sense of security and preparedness.

Review and Revision of Crisis Plans

Regular Evaluations

Collaborative crisis plans are subject to regular evaluations. Therapists engage in ongoing discussions with individuals and their support network to assess the effectiveness of the crisis plan. This involves exploring whether the identified strategies are still relevant and making adjustments based on the individual's evolving needs.

Revision in Response to Changes

Therapists guide individuals in revising their crisis plans in response to life changes or shifts in recovery progress. This may include updating contact information, modifying coping strategies or incorporating new insights gained through therapy. The ability to adapt the crisis plan ensures its continued relevance and effectiveness.

Empowering Through Collaboration in Crisis Planning

Collaborative crisis planning is a dynamic and evolving process that empowers individuals and their support networks. Therapists serve as facilitators in creating comprehensive crisis plans that are personalised, proactive and responsive to individual needs. By involving the support network, fostering shared decision-making and integrating technology and resources, collaborative crisis planning is the cornerstone of resilience in trauma recovery. This contingency approach prepares individuals for potential crises and strengthens their control and self-efficacy in the face of adversity. In the collaborative journey of crisis planning, individuals and their support networks emerge as active agents in their ongoing recovery, equipped with the tools and strategies needed to navigate challenges and thrive beyond trauma.

Navigating the Path to Healing

As we conclude this journey through the pages of this book, we recognise the depth and complexity of the topic at hand – trauma, its impact on individuals and their journeys towards healing. We've explored the intricacies of trauma, delving into the physiological, psychological and emotional dimensions. The chapters have unfolded as a guide, offering insights, strategies and collaborative approaches to foster recovery.

From understanding the nature of trauma to recognising its signs and symptoms, we've navigated the intricate landscape of the mind and body in the aftermath of distress. The exploration of coping strategies, seeking professional help and the power of narrative processing is a roadmap towards resilience. We've engaged with the cultural and social dimensions of trauma, recognising the importance of diverse narratives and the role of storytelling in the healing process.

The chapters on relapse prevention, family involvement and collaborative crisis planning underscore the significance of a supportive network in the journey to recovery. We've emphasised the need for a holistic approach, recognising the interplay of the individual within their familial, social and cultural contexts.

In the chapters on resilience, mindset and thriving, we've glimpsed the future, acknowledging that healing is not just about overcoming the past but actively shaping a meaningful and purposeful life. The narrative processing of trauma becomes a tool for empowerment, allowing individuals to move from being victims to survivors and, ultimately, thrivers.

The book serves as a guide for individuals, therapists and support networks alike. It is a testament to the strength of the human spirit, the resilience that resides within and the transformative power of collaborative healing. It is an acknowledgment that healing is not linear; it's a journey with peaks and valleys, progress and setbacks, but always moving towards growth and recovery.

As you, the reader, close these pages, remember that healing is a continuous process. Embrace the complexities of your journey, celebrate the victories and acknowledge the challenges. Seek support when needed, engage in the power of storytelling and nurture a mindset that looks towards a future filled with possibilities.

May this book stand as a companion on your path to healing — a source of knowledge, inspiration and encouragement. The journey continues, and so does the potential for growth, resilience and a life beyond the shadows of trauma.

Visit *https://mazdak.co/page/resources*
to sign up and access your free bonuses today.

References

Hanh, T.N. (2008) *The Miracle of Mindfulness*. Rider Publishing.

Herman, J. (1997) *Trauma and Recovery*. Basic Books.

Lineham, M.M. (2014) *DBT Skills Training Handouts and Worksheets*. Guilford Press.

Nestor, J. (2021) *Breath: the new science of lost art*. Penguin Life.

Reivich, K. and Shatte, A. (2003) *The Resilience Factor*. R Wyler & Co.

Schauer, M., Neuner, F., Elbert, T. (2011) *Narrative Exposure Therapy: A Short-Term Treatment for Traumatic Stress Disorders*. Hogrefe Publishing.

van der Kolk, B. (2015) *The Body Keeps the Score*. Penguin.

Young, J.E. and Klosko, J.S. (2019) *Reinventing your Life*. Scribe Publications.

www.ingramcontent.com/pod-product-compliance
Lightning Source LLC
Chambersburg PA
CBHW070405270326
41926CB00014B/2715